CAMBRIDGE PUBLIC HEALTH SERIES

UNDER THE EDITORSHIP OF

G. S. GRAHAM-SMITH, M.D. *University Lecturer in Hygiene and Secretary to the Sub-Syndicate for Tropical Medicine*

AND

J. E. PURVIS, M.A. *University Lecturer in Chemistry and Physics in their application to Hygiene and Preventive Medicine, and Secretary to the State Medicine Syndicate*

T0296188

ISOLATION HOSPITALS

ISOLATION HOSPITALS

BY

H. FRANKLIN PARSONS,
M.D. (Lond.), D.P.H. (Camb.)

SOMETIME FIRST ASSISTANT MEDICAL OFFICER OF THE LOCAL GOVERNMENT BOARD

SECOND EDITION

REVISED AND PARTLY RE-WRITTEN BY

R. BRUCE LOW, C.B.,
M.D. (Edin.), D.P.H. (Camb.)

FORMERLY SECOND ASSISTANT MEDICAL OFFICER OF THE LOCAL GOVERNMENT BOARD
AND MEDICAL OFFICER, MINISTRY OF HEALTH

CAMBRIDGE
AT THE UNIVERSITY PRESS
1922

CAMBRIDGE UNIVERSITY PRESS
Cambridge, New York, Melbourne, Madrid, Cape Town, Singapore,
São Paulo, Delhi, Dubai, Tokyo, Mexico City

Cambridge University Press
The Edinburgh Building, Cambridge CB2 8RU, UK

Published in the United States of America by Cambridge University Press, New York

www.cambridge.org
Information on this title: www.cambridge.org/9780521175975

First edition 1914
Second edition 1922
First paperback edition 2010

A catalogue record for this publication is available from the British Library

ISBN 978-0-521-17597-5 Paperback

EDITORS' PREFACE

IN view of the increasing importance of the study of public hygiene and the recognition by doctors, teachers, administrators and members of Public Health and Hygiene Committees alike that the *salus populi* must rest, in part at least, upon a scientific basis, the Syndics of the Cambridge University Press have decided to publish a series of volumes dealing with the various subjects connected with Public Health.

The books included in the Series present in a useful and handy form the knowledge now available in many branches of the subject. They are written by experts, and the authors are occupied, or have been occupied, either in investigations connected with the various themes or in their application and administration. They include the latest scientific and practical information offered in a manner which is not too technical. The bibliographies contain references to the literature of each subject which will ensure their utility to the specialist.

It has been the desire of the editors to arrange that the books should appeal to various classes of readers : and it is hoped that they will be useful to the medical profession at home and abroad, to bacteriologists and laboratory students, to municipal engineers and architects, to medical officers of health and sanitary inspectors and to teachers and administrators.

Many of the volumes will contain material which will be suggestive and instructive to members of Public Health and Hygiene Committees; and it is intended that they shall seek to influence the large body of educated and intelligent public opinion interested in the problems of public health.

January 1914.

PREFACE TO THE SECOND EDITION

A SECOND edition of *Isolation Hospitals* having been urgently demanded the whole text was carefully revised and, where necessary, portions were rewritten and brought as far as possible up to date. The part of the book which needed most amendment and alteration was that devoted to Sanatoria. These institutions, it is generally acknowledged, are still undergoing a process of evolution which in recent years has been greatly retarded by circumstances arising out of the great war. It is however expected that some advancement will shortly take place and that the construction and arrangement of Sanatoria will probably be much improved in the near future. It is therefore necessary to point out that what is now written in this work concerning Sanatoria can only be regarded in the meantime as provisional, although based upon the latest available official information. Some of the illustrations which appeared in the first edition have been suppressed as no longer being altogether up to date, and they have been replaced by others which are regarded as being more representative of present day views.

Thanks are due to Sir George Newman, K.C.B., for permission to make use of plans and memoranda belonging to the Ministry of Health; also to Dr T. Eustace Hill, O.B.E., Medical Officer of Health for the County of Durham, and to Dr H. Spurrier, Medical Superintendent of the National Sanatorium, Benenden, Kent, for permission to reproduce photographs of certain Sanatoria. Special thanks are owing to Dr A. S. MacNalty and Dr J. E. Chapman, Medical Officers of the Ministry of Health, for their kind advice and assistance in revising the section of the book which deals with Sanatoria.

R. B. L.

December, 1921

AUTHOR'S PREFACE TO FIRST EDITION

I N writing a book on Isolation Hospitals as one of the
volumes of the *Cambridge Public Health Series*, the special
aim of the author has been to produce a work which shall be of
practical use to members of local authorities, medical officers of
health, hospital superintendents and others interested in the
establishment or management of hospitals for infectious diseases;
and he hopes that the experience gained during a long official
career may have enabled him to include some useful information
and suggestions not otherwise readily obtainable. A chapter
on Sanatoria for Tuberculosis has been included in view of the
importance of this subject at the present time, when the provision of the accommodation necessary for affording "sanatorium
benefit" under the National Insurance Act, 1911, is engaging the
attention of public bodies. The matter is at present in a stage
of rapid evolution, and anything that can be written upon it
must be regarded as only provisional; but the chapter gives the
latest official pronouncements on the subject.

On subjects of controversy, such as the utility of hospital
isolation of scarlet fever, the aerial convection of infection from
small-pox hospitals, and bed-isolation in relation to the prevention of cross-infection and of "return cases," the author has
endeavoured to give a fair summary of the arguments on either
side, believing himself that the truth will probably be found to
lie somewhere between the two extreme views, or perhaps in
some altogether different and unexpected direction. He thinks,
however, that bed-isolation, whether by structural separation or
by aseptic methods of nursing, affords the most likely way out
of the difficulties and drawbacks attendant upon the hospital
treatment of infectious diseases. There is reason to believe that

in infectious diseases the primary infection is liable to have
accompanying or supervening upon it other secondary septic
infections, to which latter the severity of the resulting illness
and the occurrence of complications are largely due; that these
secondary infections may be different even where the primary
infection is the same; and that therefore every patient suffering
from an acute infectious disease should be regarded as requiring to
be isolated—more or less completely according to the nature and
stage of the disease—not only from healthy susceptible persons,
and from persons suffering from illness due to other infections
but also from other cases which are classified as being of the same
infectious disease. Similar principles explain the evil results
which have in the past been observed to follow overcrowding
and want of strict cleanliness in hospitals, whether for infectious
diseases or for surgical cases alone.

　To the complaints made from time to time with respect to
the excessive cost of isolation hospitals, the answer is that the
present high cost of maintenance of such institutions is mainly
due to the routine practice of removing to hospital all cases of
scarlet fever; that in the present mild phase of scarlet fever many
of these cases would do equally well if treated at home, and that
much saving to the rates and little detriment to the public
health would probably result if the removal of scarlet fever to
hospital were limited to exceptional cases of special urgency;
but that hospital isolation is found such a convenience by the
public that any such limitation—as indicated above—would be
likely to give rise to very grave dissatisfaction especially among
the working classes. The high cost per bed of construction of
isolation hospitals is due partly to the nature of the accommodation needed, but also largely to the difficulty of obtaining
suitable sites. Combination with other districts affords the most
feasible means of reducing the cost to small districts. Temporary hospitals of wood or iron have serious disadvantages and
their apparent cheapness is in large part illusory.

　In conclusion the author desires to express his special thanks
to Dr Newsholme, C.B., Medical Officer of the Local Government
Board, for permission to make use of notes and plans in the
possession of the Board, and to other of his former colleagues

belonging to the Local Government Board; to Dr J. S. Tew, Medical Officer of Health for the East Kent Combined District, Dr S. Barwise, County Medical Officer of Health for Derbyshire, Dr Philip Boobbyer of Nottingham, and other medical officers of health, for information and illustrations, and to Mr T. Duncombe Mann, Clerk to the Metropolitan Asylums Board. The author is also indebted to the proprietors of the *Municipal Journal* for Figs. 54 and 55, to Messrs Wilson and Stockall, Bury, Lancashire, for Figs. 24—26, Messrs Humphreys, Limited, Knightsbridge, London, for Figs. 12—23 and 28, Messrs Boulton and Paul, Norwich, for Figs. 34—38, and the Hygienic Constructions and Portable Buildings, Limited, London, for Fig. 29 and other plans.

H. F. P.

August 1913.

———————————————

The proofs of this book were being passed through the press at the time of the author's death, and the Editors of the Series were fortunately able to obtain the services of Dr R. Bruce Low, formerly of the Local Government Board, who kindly undertook the correction and completion of the whole work. The General Editors and the Syndics of the University Press desire to thank Dr Bruce Low for the great care and ample knowledge he has devoted to this service.

J. E. P.
G. S. G.-S.

21 *January* 1914.

CONTENTS

LIST OF TEXT FIGURES

CHAPTER I

HISTORICAL

It was only during the second half of the last century that the provision of means of isolation for persons affected with the infectious diseases ordinarily current in a community became recognised as the function and duty of local authorities. Many centuries earlier, indeed, provision had been made for the isolation and lodgment of persons affected with leprosy (under which name, as Hirsch considers, were probably included other affections more readily communicable from person to person than the disease to which the name of "leprosy" is now restricted) by the establishment of what were called leper-houses or "lazars" (in allusion to Lazarus the diseased beggar of the parable in St Luke's Gospel); these establishments were founded by the sovereign, by ecclesiastical bodies or by private benefactors. The first are said to have been established among the Franks in the 8th century, and at the beginning of the 13th century there were as many as 2000 in France, almost every town being obliged to build one. There were also many in England, and their former existence is sometimes commemorated in place-names, as that of Burton Lazars, Leicestershire. Their establishment seems to have been prompted not only by Christian charity but also by a belief in the contagious nature of this terrible disease, as well as by the idea of spiritual defilement associated with it, and the desire to remove the loathsome sight of its victims from the public view.

In subsequent centuries when outbreaks of plague frequently recurred in England it became the practice to erect or set apart

buildings outside the towns, called " Pest houses," for the isolation of persons suffering from plague, and perhaps other diseases
recognised as infectious. They were apparently provided by the
parishioners independently of any legal enactment. A few have
survived to our own times ; at Huntingdon, Woodbridge, Watford and Sevenoaks, an old house outside the town, bearing the
name Pest House, was in occasional use for isolation purposes at
least as recently as 1892.

According to Dr Murchison the definite establishment of
fever hospitals was the outcome of the fatal typhus epidemic
which committed such ravages at the close of the 18th century,
and the first was opened at Chester by Dr Haygarth. Liverpool, Manchester, Norwich, Hull, Dublin, London and other
towns soon followed ; and at the same time the necessity of
establishing fever wards in the old hospitals was acknowledged,
and in many cases acted on. It appears to have been the
previous practice to treat fever cases in the same wards with other
patients, a practice which continued more or less until towards
the latter part of the 19th century. The London Fever Hospital
was established in 1802, but the London Small-Pox Hospital had
been established in 1745, and the Lock Hospital for venereal
diseases in 1746. All these hospitals appear to have been established by private effort, doubtless under the influence of the great
humanitarian movement which commenced in the middle of the
18th century. The name " House of Recovery" borne by some
of these early fever hospitals indicates that the founders had in
view the relief of the individual patient rather than the protection of the community.

The Public Health Act, 1848, the first general public health
Act, contained no clause authorising the local boards of health
established under it to provide hospitals for infectious diseases.
At that date medical knowledge concerning the propagation of
the infectious fevers was less definite than it is now, and the
early sanitary reformers were inclined to look for their origin in
the universal fouling of the air, the soil, and the water-supply
which they found to exist, rather than in specific infection. It is
probable too that public opinion, which, as it was, was not
prepared for the drastic measures advocated by the first General

Board of Health, would not have sanctioned the expense of establishing isolation hospitals, or have approved any measures which savoured of interference with the liberty of the subject. It has doubtless been well on the whole for the country that the earlier efforts of sanitary reformers were directed towards promoting a condition of cleanliness unfavourable for the propagation of epidemic diseases, rather than towards combating these diseases more directly, possibly by measures akin to quarantine; but the course adopted had the disadvantage that, when the question of hospital provision by public authorities for infectious cases came to be taken up, it was done for Poor Law purposes, and was thus started on a wrong track, as a measure for the relief of necessitous individuals rather than as one for the protection of the public health, and hence many difficulties arose.

Moreover in the middle of the last century considerable difference of opinion existed among physicians upon the relative advantages of isolating fever patients, and of distributing them in the wards of a general hospital; and keen controversialists had declared on the one hand that "it would be better to have no hospitals at all than to mix cases of typhus, small-pox, and scarlet fever with patients suffering from other diseases," and on the other hand that all cases of infectious disease ought to be distributed through the wards of general hospitals and that fever hospitals and fever wards were "a crime against humanity and a disgrace to the age in which we live[1]." The circumstance that most of the nurses and other officials of fever hospitals contracted fever had produced a reaction in favour of the system of mixing the patients, and in 1842 the opinions of a number of hospital physicians in London who were consulted on the point were unanimously hostile to separate fever wards and favourable to the mixing of fever patients with others, provided the proportion was kept low.

A circular issued in 1860 on behalf of the London Fever Hospital elicited the information that of 11 London general hospitals 8 admitted a limited number of fever cases among the

---

[1] Murchison, *A Treatise on the Continued Fevers of Great Britain*, 1862, 2nd edition, 1873, Chapter 8.

general cases, while 3 admitted no cases of fever.   Of 20
hospitals in the provinces, 9 refused to admit fever patients.
6 admitted them into separate wards and only 5 distributed
them among the general patients.   In every one of 4 Scotch
hospitals there were separate fever wards.   Of 5 Irish hospitals,
1 was limited to fever cases; in 3 there were separate fever
wards, and in only 1 were the fever cases distributed among the
general patients.   In most of the large towns of Ireland there
was a special hospital for the treatment of infectious diseases.
The larger extent to which fever-cases were admitted into the
London hospitals was due partly to the desire of affording to
students the opportunity of studying cases of fever and partly
to the circumstance that a large proportion of the fever cases in
London were of enteric fever, a disease which does not spread
in the wards like typhus.

At that time typhus was still, and relapsing fever had been
until recently, frequent in London and other large towns, and
epidemics of both diseases occurred from time to time.   In the
London Fever Hospital up to the close of 1861 there was no
classification of the patients, and cases of typhus were treated in
the same wards with cases of enteric fever, scarlet fever and
other diseases.   After 1861 the typhus cases were separately
treated, but the classification was often broken through in consequence of the crowded state of the hospital.   Separate wards
for scarlet fever seem also to have been instituted about the
same time, and small-pox was not admitted, the need for
separate treatment of this disease being more generally recognised.

Dr Murchison pointed out that, as it was admitted that
where typhus patients were mixed with others there was danger
of the disease spreading if the proportion of typhus cases
exceeded 1 in 6, there was need for fever hospitals during
epidemics to receive the surplus.   " Every one who has paid any
attention to the subject admits that even in seasons when the
disease is not epidemic, patients with typhus ought not to be
treated in their own crowded houses where the fever would
inevitably spread, and it is clear that they must be removed,
either to fever hospitals or special fever wards, or be interspersed

among the other patients of a general hospital." The latter
plan appeared to Dr Murchison objectionable on the following
grounds:

1. There are numberless instances where typhus has spread
in general wards, notwithstanding the most careful precautions,
and where the proportion of cases has not exceeded 1 in 6, or
where it has spread from even a single case.

[He quoted many instances.]

2. The two objections usually urged against fever hospitals
and fever wards, that owing to the concentration of the poison
the mortality among the patients themselves and the danger of
the fever spreading are increased are contradicted by facts.

[During the first 6 months of 1862, 1107 cases of typhus were under treatment
in the London Fever Hospital of which 232 died, a case mortality of 20·95 per
cent. During the same period 343 cases of typhus were treated in general
hospitals in London, and of this number 80 died or 23·32 per cent. The
1080 cases (1107 – 27) admitted into the Fever Hospital communicated the
disease to 27 other persons, of whom 8 died, *i.e.* 1 person took the fever
for every 40 admitted, and 1 died for every 135 admitted. The 272 cases
admitted into the general hospitals communicated the disease to 71 persons,
of whom 21 died; or 1 person caught the fever for every 3·8 cases admitted,
and 1 died for every 12·9 cases admitted. In the 4 years 1862–5 1 person took
typhus for every 5 typhus patients admitted into the general hospitals, but only
1 for every 67 admitted into the London Fever Hospital; 1 person died of
typhus for every 14 admitted into the former but only 1 for every 326 admitted
into the latter.]

3. The maladies for which patients are ordinarily admitted
into general hospitals predispose them to contract typhus on
exposure to the contagion, and to have it in a severe and fatal
form.

4. The ventilation which is universally admitted to be
necessary for preventing typhus spreading in a general ward is
injurious to patients suffering from many diseases, such as
nephritis, acute rheumatism, bronchitis, etc.

5. In a fever hospital or fever wards it will be always
possible to obtain a staff of officials seasoned by a previous
attack of typhus, or of an age at which it is not very likely to be
fatal, which it would be impossible to obtain for general
hospitals.

Dr Murchison's experience led him to the following conclusions as to the proper mode of dealing with fever patients.

1.   Cases of enteric fever may be distributed in the wards of a general hospital with impunity.

2.   Cases of typhus and of relapsing fever ought never to be treated in a ward with other patients; even in no larger a proportion than 1 in 6 there is a danger of these diseases spreading.

3.   There is no evidence that in a well ventilated fever hospital the mortality from continued fevers is greater than in a general hospital.

4.   In proportion to the number of cases of typhus treated the danger of the disease spreading is much less on the plan of isolation than on that of mixing.

5.   Fever hospitals are absolutely necessary in all large towns liable to epidemics of typhus, and they ought to be provided with the means of rapid extension by the erection of temporary buildings of wood or iron in the event of an epidemic breaking out.

6.   In all general hospitals there ought, when possible, to be arrangements for the treatment of contagious fevers, otherwise many acute cases, not contagious, are practically excluded. But the contagious cases ought not to be interspersed through the general wards; they ought to be isolated in separate wards, or better in a detached building.

7.   In every fever hospital, typhus, relapsing fever, enteric fever and scarlatina ought to be treated in distinct wards; but there can be no objection to the many cases of acute non-contagious diseases, constantly sent by mistake to fever hospitals, being treated in the same wards with enteric fever.

A view contrary to that of Dr Murchison was expressed in an elaborate report by Dr J. S. Bristowe and Mr T. Holmes, on "The Hospitals of the United Kingdom" included with the 6th Report of the Medical Officer of the Privy Council, 1863. The reporters said: "The system of separate fever wards is one which deserves very careful consideration. It is intimately connected with the question of risk of contagion; and this, there can be no doubt, varies very greatly for different diseases. Thus if small-pox be received into any part of a general hospital, there is much danger of its affecting patients even in other parts. In the Scotch hospitals, and in several of our English hospitals, small-pox appears to be admitted, though only in scattered cases, into the fever wards, or into separate wards adjacent to them; in some cases however it has spread in the hospital. On the whole, as far as our present experience goes, it appears unjustifiable to expose patients in a general hospital to the risk of having cases of small-pox among them. It is otherwise with the other exanthemata; scarlet fever is received at many of the London Hospitals, and as far as we know (having had long personal experience of two of them) without any detriment; nor does it appear certain that typhoid has manifested any tendency to spread among the patients. With typhus the case is otherwise.

" In the case of separate fever wards however or fever houses, the evidence is not of this negative description. Sad experience has shown how extremely dangerous such places are to the medical and other attendants on the patients and to the patients themselves. During the short time we have spent upon this enquiry, and among the comparatively few hospitals which comprise a separate fever house or fever wards, we have visited no less than three in which the resident medical officer had just died of fever caught in the wards, while in others the house surgeon or other residents had been attacked but had recovered.

" It seems then, on a review of the evidence that we possess, that if in a general hospital fevers of all kinds be scattered about in the wards there is some risk of the spread of fever to the patients; if they be collected into separate wards there is great danger to the medical attendants. In either case the nurses will be in danger, and of course in much greater danger under the latter system."

" When typhus fever is so prevalent that, if it were indiscriminately admitted, the wards would become crowded with it, it appears that even the best constructed hospitals will be poisoned by it, and become unfit for the purposes of a general hospital. Otherwise, that is when the proportion of cases of fever to general cases is small, there seems no great risk in admitting them if the hospital is well ventilated, and the beds a sufficient distance apart, and if patients who are well enough to go about are carefully kept away from the fever beds. We believe that if our county hospitals were of perfect construction, a moderate number of fever cases (say one or two in each ward according to their size) might be admitted without danger, and that this plan would be far preferable to that of special fever wards by which so many valuable lives have already been sacrificed. But in order that fevers may be safely received the general arrangements and ventilation of the hospital must be very different from those which we have described at many country hospitals, where no doubt the more prudent course has been adopted in excluding these diseases altogether. It must be remembered however that the cases must be treated somewhere, and if the hospital is well constructed it ought to be a far more fit place for the treatment of disease than a poorhouse infirmary or a crowded cottage."

"The treatment of contagious diseases no doubt involves risk. No doubt such diseases if taken into any hospital, general or special, will occasionally spread but will they not spread if the patient is left at home? And is not the spread of such fevers due in part to the fact that so many of our hospitals, particularly in small country towns, shrink from the performance of their most serious duty, viz., that of treating the acutest forms of disease? If it be replied that in such case separate fever-houses should be added to the hospital, we would remark that such fever-houses are often found to be almost superfluous, from the small number of patients who apply at times when fever is not epidemic, and that when this is the case a valuable portion of the hospital is kept unoccupied. But that the hospital should have the power of treating acute disease is the first requisite, and for this it is necessary that no rule should exist excluding fevers."

"Our own impression leads us to believe that scattering the cases is the safest course if the hospital be spacious and the applications not too numerous. We repeat that for the safe reception of fever cases large well ventilated wards and beds well removed from each other are essential."

The reporters' view was upheld by Sir John Simon who considered that rules which prohibited the admission of cases of contagious disease into general hospitals implied the dereliction of a hospital's most important functions. " I cannot conceive," he said, " any cases having more claim to hospital treatment than those cases of typhoid, and sometimes typhus fever, which the rules would rigidly exclude. To leave such cases in the ill-provided homes of the poor is not only to withhold the assistance of the charity from persons in very urgent need of the best attainable medical treatment, but it further involves as an almost necessary result, that the disease shall continue its ravages in the family, and perhaps greatly beyond the family, which it has attacked." He also alluded to the indirect effect of such a regulation in excluding other large classes of acute disease which pre-eminently claimed hospital treatment. It had been found by the reporters that the admission or non-admission of infectious disease practically regulated in no small degree the admission of other acute medical diseases. Where a regulation that no cases of fever be admitted was enforced not only did actual fever cases cease to apply, but all those cases which the lay public might ordinarily regard as fevers, and those in which a skilled medical practitioner might hesitate for the moment to commit himself to an opinion ceased also to apply. The number of cases of other acute and serious diseases which might be mistaken for fever was illustrated by the experience of the London Fever Hospital in 1861, in which year out of 646 cases admitted, 473 were of typhus, typhoid, scarlet fever and measles, and 173, or 26·8 per cent. were cases of non-infectious acute disease[1]. The mortality among these non-infectious cases was 28·3 per cent. while the general mortality of the hospital for the year was only 18·2 per cent. (This would apparently make the mortality of the infectious cases only 14·6 per cent.) The most numerous causes of death were phthisis or acute tuberculosis, acute hydrocephalus,

[1] In the Metropolitan Asylums Board's fever hospitals the proportion of cases admitted on a mistaken diagnosis to total admissions was in 1910 11·3 per cent. and in 1911 10·6 per cent. Many of the cases so admitted were however of infectious diseases other and less serious than those notified, *e.g.* chicken-pox and rubella, and others had no obvious disease. The mortality among these cases in 1911 was 5·5 per cent. while among the ordinary infectious cases it was 6·72 per cent. The most frequent causes of death were pneumonia, broncho-pneumonia and tuberculous meningitis.

pneumonia and diseases of the heart and kidneys. In hospitals from which infectious diseases were by rule excluded the medical cases which applied for admission were purely chronic and for the most part trivial.

The provision of hospitals for infectious diseases by public authorities, and the virtual extinction of typhus fever have put an end to these old controversies, though they still have their moral. At the present time the practice of receiving infectious cases into general hospitals—even into detached buildings, as at some hospitals mentioned in Dr Thorne's report in 1882—has almost ceased, though enteric fever—a disease now recognised as being more readily communicable from person to person than it was considered to be in Dr Murchison's time—is still sometimes admitted, and occasionally diphtheria, especially cases urgently requiring operation. It is desirable, however, as pointed out by Dr Murchison, that general hospitals should possess some small wards suitably placed for the isolation of infectious cases which may be admitted under a mistaken diagnosis or in the stage of incubation; as the patient may not be able to bear removal to the public isolation hospital, or it may be desired to continue some surgical or other special treatment needed for the disease for which the patient was originally admitted.

Workhouse Infirmaries. Prior to 1866, except for such cases as could be admitted into the comparatively few fever or small-pox hospitals which then existed, or into general hospitals, the only places into which persons suffering from infectious diseases who were without proper accommodation in their own homes could be removed were the workhouse infirmaries. Here they were mixed with other patients, to the danger of the latter; and were nursed and attended to by pauper nurses, commonly feeble old men and women, ignorant of nursing and too often vicious and neglectful.

An Act was passed in 1790 "To impower Justices and other persons to visit parish workhouses or poorhouses and examine and certify the state and condition of the Poor therein to the Quarter Sessions." The preamble of this Act says: "Whereas the laws now in being for the regulating parish workhouses or poorhouses have been found in certain instances deficient and ineffectual, especially when the poor in such houses are afflicted with contagious or infectious diseases, in which cases particular attention to their lodging, diet, cloathing, bedding and medicines is requisite." If in such visitation any of the poor should be found afflicted with any contagious or infectious disease an application might be made to the justices of the division and any two justices might make an order for the immediate procuring of medical or other assistance, or of sufficient or proper food, or for the separation or removal of such poor as shall be afflicted with any contagious or infectious disease.

In the early "sixties" of the 19th century the public mind was aroused by a remarkable series of articles which appeared in the *Lancet* containing the investigations of Dr F. Anstie and Mr Ernest Hart into the condition of the London workhouse infirmaries, extended subsequently to those outside London. The grave charges made against these institutions were confirmed by a report made to the Poor Law Board in 1866 by Dr Edward Smith, "on the conditions of the infirmaries and sick wards of the metropolitan workhouses and their arrangements." The result was the passing of the Metropolitan Poor Law Act 1867 which gave to the Poor Law Board the power to combine into districts the numerous metropolitan Unions and separate parishes previously maintaining their own poor, for the purpose of establishing asylums for the reception and relief of the sick and infirm, and under this power the whole of these Unions and parishes were combined into a single district, for the purpose of providing hospitals for the reception and relief of poor persons chargeable to any Union or parish in the district who might be infected with or suffering from fever or small-pox. The Metropolitan Asylums Board, thus constituted purely for poor law ends, has ultimately become the hospital authority for London for public health purposes, as will be narrated more fully later on in Chapter XVI.

Outside London the policy of the Poor Law Board seems to have been to secure the provision in connection with workhouses of suitable detached fever wards, and ward blocks for infectious cases more or less up to the standard of the time were erected at many workhouses. See Chapter XV.

The Poor Law Amendment Act of 1869 gave power for the detention in the workhouse of any poor person therein suffering from bodily disease of an infectious or contagious character on the report of the medical officer that such person was not in a proper state to leave the workhouse without danger to himself or others.

It was however soon found, both in London and elsewhere, that the provision of fever wards under the Poor Law, even if separate buildings, by no means fulfilled the needs of the community. Admission to such buildings was by law restricted to persons who were destitute, and was obtainable only by order of a relieving officer; it also constituted the person admitted, or chargeable for the patient, a pauper, entailing loss of civil privileges including the parliamentary vote. These civil disabilities were later removed by legislation, but nevertheless, the association of the hospital with the workhouse by its position and administration rendered its use distasteful to the independent artisan class or to others of higher social positions who might require removal to hospital on the ground that they could not be safely isolated or efficiently nursed at their own homes. Such persons are much more numerous than those who when suffering from infectious illness would require relief on the ground of destitution, and this is especially the case in districts where wages are comparatively high. In such districts the families containing children and young persons of the ages at which infectious diseases are most frequent are usually above the pauper line, and the recipients of outdoor relief are mostly old and infirm persons of ages little susceptible to such diseases. Further, as it was found that there was a liability of spread of infectious diseases, especially small-pox, to other inmates of the workhouse, even when the patients were treated in a separate building, if the administration were in common, it became the policy to exclude from the fever wards even pauper cases from the outside, reserving the wards solely for cases of infectious disease originating in the workhouse.

For these reasons it often happened that there was no place to which a patient urgently requiring removal to hospital could be admitted, while at the same time there was suitable accommodation for cases of infectious disease at the workhouse, provided at considerable cost, but lying idle and rarely used. Sometimes in circumstances of special urgency a patient might be admitted under a lax interpretation of the rule as to destitution, or by granting the relief on loan, but there were objections to these courses; and eventually the course which found favour, outside London, was to remove infectious cases from the workhouse, giving the sanitary authority the power to provide hospitals to which infectious patients from all classes of the population might be sent.

In 1879 an Act was passed[1] which contained a clause for facilitating the transfer of workhouse infectious hospitals in rural districts to the sanitary authority.

Cholera Hospitals. By §§ 5, 6 of the Diseases Prevention Act, 1855, "whenever any part of England appears to be threatened, or is affected by any formidable epidemic, endemic, or contagious disease" the General Board of Health, if so authorised by an Order of the Privy Council, were empowered to issue directions and regulations "for guarding against the spread of disease and affording to persons afflicted by, or threatened with such epidemic, endemic or contagious diseases, such medical aid and such accommodation as might be required." The powers of the General Board of Health were subsequently vested in the Privy Council, and by §§ 130 and 134, Public Health Act, 1875, in the Local Government Board[2]. By § 3 (1) of the Ministry of Health Act, 1919, all the powers and duties of the Local Government Board in this and other respects were transferred to the Minister of Health.

In July 1866, following on the appearance of epidemic cholera in London, Orders in Council were issued, putting in force throughout England the above provisions of the Diseases

[1] Poor Law Act, 1879, § 14. In view of the changes effected by the Local Government Act, 1894, this section is no longer available for the purpose.

[2] In view of the use of the word "endemic" the powers conferred under these sections, which were formerly regarded as having reference only to exotic diseases, have in recent years been found capable of wide and useful extension in dealing with the prevalent indigenous diseases of the country. Thus it is under these sections that the recent Tuberculosis Orders have been issued. This course affords a means of rendering a disease compulsorily notifiable without bringing it under what might be inappropriate provisions of other Acts which would be applicable to it if it were included among those notifiable under the Infectious Diseases (Notification) Acts.

Prevention Act, 1855, and providing that where the medical
officer of health or the medical adviser so recommended the
board or vestry should with as much dispatch as practicable
provide fit and proper accommodation for the reception of such
patients as have no home, or cannot be properly treated at home
and may with advantage to themselves be removed, and further
that if cholera or choleraic diarrhoea existed in any dwelling
whereof the medical practitioner reported that the sick and
healthy cannot therein be properly separated the board or vestry
should forthwith cause adequate accommodation to be procured
for the reception of the healthy.

Under these Orders several cholera hospitals were established
both in the metropolis and in the provinces, and some of these
hospitals after the danger of epidemic cholera had passed
were maintained by the local authorities for the reception of
cases of the infectious fevers of ordinary occurrence in their
districts.

By the Sanitary Act, 1866, § 37, power was given to local
authorities to provide hospitals:

"The Sewer Authority" (*i.e.* in urban districts the Town
Council, or Local Board) "or in the metropolis the Nuisance
Authority" (*i.e.* the Commissioners of Sewers and the Vestries
or District Boards) "may provide for the use of the inhabitants
within its district hospitals or temporary places for the reception
of the sick.

"Such authority may itself build such hospitals or places of
reception, or make contracts for the use of any existing hospital
or part of an hospital or for the temporary use of any place for
the reception of the sick.

"It may enter into any agreement with any person or body
of persons having the management of any hospital for the
reception of the sick inhabitants of its district on payment by
the Sewer Authority of such annual or other sums as may be
agreed upon.

"Two or more authorities having respectively the power to
provide separate hospitals may combine in providing a common
hospital, and all expenses incurred by such authorities in providing such hospital shall be deemed to be expenses incurred by

them respectively in carrying into effect the purposes of this Act."

In the Public Health Act, 1875, § 131, this provision was repeated in a modified form:

"Any local authority may provide for the use of the inhabitants of their district hospitals or temporary places for the reception of the sick, and for that purpose may—

"Themselves build such hospitals or places of reception ; or

"Contract for the use of any such hospital or part of a hospital or place of reception ; or

"Enter into any agreement with any person having the management of any hospital, for the reception of the sick inhabitants of their district, on payment of such annual or other sum as may be agreed on.

"Two or more local authorities may combine in providing a common hospital."

It is to be noted that the sick inhabitants for whose use hospitals may be provided are not only those suffering from infectious diseases. In a few places under special local conditions the local authorities have provided hospitals for accident cases or for seamen suffering from non-infectious diseases, and at Widnes and Barry the Local Government Board have sanctioned loans for the erection of such hospitals.

The powers of local authorities to provide hospitals have however chiefly been employed in securing accommodation for cases of infectious disease, and at first they were most frequently exercised in establishing temporary hospitals on the occurrence of formidable epidemics and especially of outbreaks of small-pox.

The replies to a circular letter issued by the Local Government Board in 1879 showed that at that time, out of a total of 1593 sanitary authorities in England and Wales, 296 (viz. 192 urban, 87 rural, and 17 port authorities) possessed means of some sort or other for the isolation of infectious diseases : but the hospital provision was in many cases such in name only, being rarely or never used, or was available only for one disease, usually small-pox.

In 1882 a very valuable report was made to the Local

Government Board by Dr (afterwards Sir Richard) Thorne Thorne "On the use and influence of Hospitals for Infectious Diseases." The first part of the report contained a general summary of the conclusions at which Dr Thorne had arrived respecting the construction, management and conditions of use-fulness of isolation hospitals; and the second part contained descriptions of the several hospitals visited by him in the course of his inquiry. This report long remained the standard work of reference on the subject, and was reprinted in 1901, with a preface, signed by the Board's then Medical Officer, Sir W. H. Power, F.R.S., embodying the Board's later experience up to that date[1].

Dr Thorne pointed out that the most useful function of a hospital was to receive the initial cases of an infectious disease which might occur in a locality or household, in order, by their prompt isolation, to prevent its further spread, and that in order to fulfil this function the hospital must be properly designed and must be erected beforehand and kept in readiness. He said "The suitability of the hospital buildings is to a large extent dependent upon the circumstances under which they have been erected. If a hospital is hurriedly built under the influence of panic it is often not ready for occupation until the immediate cause of its erection has passed by; it provides accommodation of a very indifferent sort; it fails, almost without exception, to meet the permanent requirements of the district, even when in amount it turns out to be more than the district needs; and thus the object of the hospital as a part of the sanitary defences of the district is often attained in a very imperfect manner and at a needlessly large cost.

"On the other hand the hospitals which have been erected during non-epidemic periods, and with a view of preventing epidemics by having in actual readiness means for the isolation of first cases of infectious disease, afford as a rule excellent examples of the kind of isolation-provision which all sanitary authorities should possess, and this report will give plentiful examples of their success in their intended object."

[1] A later report on "Isolation Hospitals," by Dr H. F. Parsons, was issued by the Local Government Board in 1912.

In the preface to the re-issue of 1901, it was pointed out that the general conclusions in the first part of Sir R. Thorne's report still for the most part held good, needing but little modification or addition, but that the local hospital reports in the second part, though still of use as a record of experience, did not afford models which could be usefully followed at the present day, or show the amount or character of the hospital accommodation now possessed by the districts there mentioned ; most of the districts referred to in the report as having hospitals of a temporary character, having since replaced them by permanent buildings.

A Parliamentary return issued in 1895 showed that out of 1653 extra-metropolitan sanitary authorities existing in England and Wales at the end of 1892, 631 had at that date provided, alone or jointly with other authorities, some kind of hospital accommodation for infectious diseases, as against 296 in 1879. During the seven years 1893—9, 334 loans for hospital purposes —not all however relating to newly established or different hospitals—were sanctioned by the Local Government Board, while many other authorities provided themselves with hospital accommodation without the aid of loans, either by the erection of buildings—often indeed of a more or less temporary or make-shift character—or by entering into agreements for the use of hospitals belonging to other districts.

Combination of districts for the purpose of joint hospital provision was also more freely resorted to, and the number of Joint Hospital Boards, which was 32 in 1892, increased to 51 at the end of 1900 and 83 in 1910, while other districts combined in a less formal manner.

Concurrent powers of hospital provision and combination of districts were given by the Isolation Hospitals Act, 1893 (amended by that of 1901), which placed in the hands of County Councils powers for the formation of hospital districts and promotion of isolation hospitals. In some counties these powers have been freely exercised, and up to the end of 1909, some 70 Joint Hospital Committees had been formed by Orders of the County Councils.

But about the end of the last century a reaction against hospitals for infectious diseases set in, and their provision and use were criticized from two points of view—financial and medical. Local authorities complained of the alleged excessive and increasing cost of the erection of isolation hospitals and of the burden of their upkeep; while from the medical point of view it was contended that they had failed to fulfil the hopes, alleged to have been held out by their promoters, that by their means infectious diseases could be " stamped out "; that on the contrary the prevalence of these diseases had not been diminished, and the aggregation of cases in hospital had introduced new dangers, as of "cross infection" and "return cases"; and it was said, in rhetoric as heated as that used by the disputants over the hospital isolation of typhus, that "the infective sick are herded like dumb driven cattle in pest-houses miscalled isolation hospitals."

In some degree both of these objections, medical and financial, had their origin in the increased extent to which hospital isolation of scarlet fever had come into practice. In 1882 Sir R. Thorne said, "Scarlet fever has only rarely been an immediate cause of hospital provision, and this notwithstanding the fact that the mortality it occasions has been so greatly in excess of that resulting from small-pox." But during the course of the next two decades scarlet fever had come to be looked on as the disease, *par excellence*, requiring hospital isolation. Some hospitals were exclusively reserved for it, cases of diphtheria and enteric fever, though more urgently requiring hospital treatment, not being admitted ; and in most isolation hospitals the cases of scarlet fever formed the great majority of those treated. In some districts too the policy was to endeavour to get every case of scarlet fever, or at any rate as large a proportion of the cases as possible, into hospital ; and on occasion of an epidemic, this sometimes led, where the amount of accommodation was insufficient, to over-crowding of the hospital and breakdown of the arrangements, with detriment to the welfare of the patients and to the health of the nurses. During the decades in question owing to the milder type commonly assumed by scarlet fever, the mortality from that disease had greatly diminished, but its prevalence had not diminished in like proportion[1], so that it was sometimes considered that in paying large amounts for the hospital treatment of cases of scarlet fever local authorities were not getting value for their money. The prolonged infectiousness of scarlet fever, sometimes after apparently complete recovery, involves long detention in hospital; leads to provision of specially arranged wards with a view to prevent cross-infection ; and sometimes gives rise to fresh cases ("return cases") after the return of the convalescent to his home ; it thus tends to render the hospital treatment of that disease costly, and to give rise to incidents which are a source of dissatisfaction.

One cause for the increased cost of isolation hospitals was of course the increased standard of efficiency which had come to be desired by local authorities and the public as the result of experience of their use. Not only was it found that, in the words of Sir R. Thorne, "people did not dread scarlatina enough to let their relatives and children be taken away to a tarred shed of repulsive aspect, such as had sufficed for the district hospital when small-pox was in question," but also that the earlier erected permanent hospitals were deficient in important respects, such as cubic space in wards, means for the separation of different diseases, accommodation for an adequate staff, laundry and other appliances, and fencing. Objections to hospitals for infectious diseases in or near towns often led to their being erected in isolated situations where public services, such as sewers, and water and gas mains were not at hand ; and the provision of drainage, water supply and lighting, whether by long connections with distant mains or by separate installations for the hospital itself, added largely to the cost of building. In the latter years of the last century, too, there was a great increase in the cost of

[1] During the last four decades the death-rate from scarlet fever in England and Wales has been as follows :

Period	1871—80	1881—90	1891—1900	1901—10
Average annual death rate per 1000 persons living	·72	·34	·16	·11

During the same periods the case-mortality among scarlet fever patients in the hospitals of the Metropolitan Asylums Board per 100 patients admitted has been

Period	1871—80	1881—90	1891—1900	1901—10
Case-mortality	12·1	10·1	4·9	3·0

building, partly due to a rise in the price of building materials but principally to a rise of wages in the building trades, an increased daily wage being conjoined with a day's work of fewer hours, and a restricted output of work per hour. It is stated that while in 1859 a rod of stock brickwork in mortar had cost approximately £12. 10s., of which £2 was for labour, in 1875 it cost £15, of which £3. 5s. was for labour, and in 1904 £16. 10s., of which £5. 10s. was for labour. Thus while hospitals, considered good in their day, built between 1885 and 1890 had cost from £164 to £309 per bed, those built at the beginning of the present century cost usually between £350 and £500 per bed.

These costs are based on cost per bed for a complete hospital at the time when the first edition of this book was issued (1914). It will be recognised that since then, owing to the great European war, conditions have entirely changed and that, in consequence, a time of considerable fluctuation in prices of building material, fittings, labour and transport, has arisen, making it impossible in the circumstances to indicate the present, even probable, cost. But there is evidence now (1921) that a reduction is already taking place in the price of material, etc., and it is probable that there may soon be a return to something like pre-war prices.

The report on "Isolation Hospitals," issued by the Local Government Board in 1912, contained some suggestions for reducing the cost of erection of isolation hospitals; but from the nature of the case, an efficient hospital for infectious disease must necessarily be a costly building, as compared with other public institutions, if the comparison is made on the basis of cost per bed.

The provision of isolation hospitals by local authorities in England and Wales is permissive, and the Local Government Board[1] have no power to compel the erection of a hospital, except in so far as this may be done by Regulations under §§ 130 or 134, P. H. Act, 1875. In Scotland, however, it is provided by § 66 of the Public Health (Scotland) Act, 1897, that any local authority may, and if required by the Local Government Board, shall, provide, furnish and maintain for the use of the inhabitants of their district, suffering from infectious disease, hospitals temporary or permanent.

During the period which has elapsed since the commencement of the present century a movement has sprung up for the pro-

[1] Now the Ministry of Health.

vision of sanatoria for the treatment of consumption (pulmonary tuberculosis) in its early and curable stages by the open air method. As in the case of fever hospitals the earliest of such sanatoria were established by private enterprise or charity, but their provision was subsequently taken up by a few local authorities, and it is now receiving much attention in view of the enactment of the National Insurance Act, 1911. See Chapter XVIII.

BIBLIOGRAPHY

Hirsch. Handbook of Geographical and Historical Pathology. New Sydenham Society's Translation. 1881. Art. Leprosy.

Newman, Sir George. The history of the decline and final extinction of Leprosy as an endemic disease in the British Islands. London. 1896.

Simon, Sir John. English Sanitary Institutions. London. 1890.

Murchison, Charles, M.D. A treatise on Continued Fevers of Great Britain. 2nd edition. 1873.

Sixth Report of Medical Officer of the Privy Council. 1863. Containing Report by Dr J. S. Bristowe and Mr Timothy Holmes on "The Hospitals of the United Kingdom."

Annual Report of Metropolitan Asylums Board. 1911.

Copnall, H. H. The Law relating to Infectious Diseases and Hospitals. Hadden, Best & Co. London. 1899.

Lancet Commission on Metropolitan Workhouse Infirmaries. 1865.

Poor Law Board. Reports of Dr Edward Smith and Dr Markham on condition of Metropolitan Workhouse Infirmaries. 1866.

Supplement to 10th Annual Report of L.G.B. 1882. [C. 3290.] Containing Report by Board's Medical Officer, Sir G. Buchanan.

    *Report on the use and influence of Hospitals for Infectious Diseases, by Dr (afterwards Sir R.) Thorne Thorne.

    *Report on the influence of the Fulham Small-pox hospital on the neighbourhood surrounding it, by Mr (afterwards Sir W. H.) Power, F.R.S.

Reprint of Sir R. Thorne's Report on the use and influence of Hospitals for Infectious Diseases. 1901. With preface by Board's Medical Officer, Sir W. H. Power.

*Parsons, H. Franklin. Report to Local Government Board on "Isolation Hospitals." 1912. [C. 6342.] Containing Memorandum by B. T. Kitchin, F.R.I.B.A., the Board's Architect, on cost of Hospitals.

*Report of the Royal Commission on Small-Pox and Fever Hospitals. 1882. [C. 3314.]

*Parliamentary Return. Sanitary Districts (Accommodation for Infectious Diseases). 1895.

Marriott, E. D. Scarlet Fever: the case against Hospital Isolation. The passing of the Isolation Hospital. Sanitary Record, 1900.

Millard, C. Killick (M.O.H. Leicester). See Bibliography to Chapter II.

Robertson and McKendrick. Public Health Law. (Livingstone, Edinburgh. 1912.)

Bulstrode, H. Timbrell. Report to the L.G.B. on Sanatoria for Consumption
    and certain other aspects of the Tuberculosis question. 1908. [C. 3657.]
Garnett, J. H. The hospital isolation of Enteric Fever. Public Health, July,
    1896. (Gives figures of cases treated in general hospitals.)
    N.B. As references to the works marked * will be frequent in the biblio-
graphy of subsequent chapters they will for the sake of brevity be referred to as
    Thorne, Hospital Report and reprint.   Report of Hospitals Commission.
    Power, Fulham Hospital Report.   1882.
    Parsons, Hospital Report.   Hospital Return. 1895.

CHAPTER II

UTILITY OF ISOLATION HOSPITALS

THE uses of a hospital for infectious diseases are :

1. The cure or relief of persons suffering from such diseases.
2. The separation of such persons from the rest of the com-
    munity with a view to prevent the spread of disease.
3. To obviate the disabilities, inconveniences and pecuniary
    losses which the presence of infectious sickness might
    entail.

The above order seems to be that in which the usefulness of
the several functions has in the course of time come to be recognised by public opinion.

A fourth use might be added, for the increasing variety of
diseases already being treated in isolation hospitals makes the
development of clinical research a necessary addition to them.
It is, alike, in the interest of the Community, the State and the
training of future Practitioners of Medicine, that a time should
come when the isolation hospital will become an institute of
Research for the elucidation of the unsolved problems relating
to the various kinds of communicable disease.

1. The primary function of a hospital of any kind is to furnish
sick persons with the housing and accommodation, food, nursing
and medical attendance which their circumstances require, and,
generally, to place them under conditions conducive to their
recovery. Whatever other uses a hospital for infectious diseases
may serve, it must not be forgotten that its first duty is to the
patients. Thus it is not right, for the sake of removing sources
of infection from the community, to overcrowd the hospital to
the detriment of the patients in it, or to expose them to danger

of infection from diseases other than those from which they were already suffering when admitted.

2. The provision of hospitals for infectious disease has, since the date when it became a function of the local sanitary authorities, been advocated especially as a measure of sanitary defence, in order that by the isolation of the first cases of an infectious disease its further spread in the locality or household invaded may be prevented ; and there can be no question that the timely isolation of an initial case is often followed by no further spread; but it must be admitted that the usefulness of an isolation hospital in arresting an outbreak of infectious disease at an early stage is more obvious than its influence in extinguishing a developed epidemic, or in reducing the endemic prevalence of a disease in a community. The routine removal to hospital of a large proportion of the scarlet fever cases occurring in a town has not, where it has been practised, effected any very notable diminution in the prevalence of the disease, and the practice is continued rather because it is demanded by the public on grounds of convenience. The householder desires to be relieved by the removal of the patient of the irksome precautions, prolonged quarantine, exclusion of children from school, interference with business, and other inconveniences which the presence of scarlet fever in his family involves ; and where, as is now usually the case in such places, treatment in a public isolation hospital is free, he may regard the money spent through the rates for the upkeep for the hospital as an expense which it is worth while to incur by way of insurance. Another influence in favour of isolation hospitals is the desire of medical men in private practice to be relieved of the duty of attending on cases of infectious disease ; a duty which might cause danger or alarm to their other patients.

It is sometimes complained that isolation hospitals have not fulfilled the prediction alleged to have been made by their advocates, that by their means infectious diseases would be " stamped out " ; it is not clear, however, that such a prediction was ever made by any responsible sanitarian and the expression does not appear to occur in any report or memorandum issued by the late Local Government Board. But it may be remarked that the

infectious diseases for which hospital accommodation was at
first most often provided, viz. cholera, small-pox and typhus,
have now become extinct, at least as endemic diseases, in most
parts of Great Britain, although no doubt other things besides
hospital isolation have had much to do with their decline.
Still, when outbreaks of small-pox or typhus do occur hospital
isolation is found indispensable for dealing with them. The
evils too which, as mentioned in the first chapter, were foreseen
by the opponents of special fever hospitals as likely to arise
from the aggregation of typhus cases have not come to pass.
Even scarlet fever itself, a disease which has similarly been
asserted to be rendered more severe by the aggregation of cases
in hospital, has shown a marked diminution of mortality, the
death-rates per million persons living in England and Wales
during successive periods of five years having been:

1871—75, 759;	1896—1900, 135;
1876—80, 680;	1901—5, 126;
1881—85, 436;	1906—10, 86;
1886—90, 241;	1911—15, 61.
1891—95, 182;	

Thus the death-rate from scarlet fever is now only about
a twelfth of what it was 50 years ago, and it may be remarked
that this diminution in the death-rate from scarlet fever has
taken place concurrently with an increase in the opportunities
for the propagation of infection which might be expected to have
tended in the opposite direction. Compulsory education, which
since 1870 has become more and more completely enforced, has
led to the aggregation of children of susceptible age daily in
public elementary schools. The progressive urbanisation of the
population has led to a large proportion of working-class families
in towns living in houses sublet to two or more families instead
of in self-contained cottages. There has been a greatly increased
use of public conveyances, such as trains, trams and omnibuses,
especially by the working class, and assemblages of various
kinds are more frequent and bring together larger numbers. In
all these ways the opportunities for the spread of infection of
a disease such as scarlet fever have been multiplied.

That the death-rate from scarlet fever has declined, under

circumstances which might be thought to tend to its increase, cannot however be ascribed in any large measure to the protection against contracting the disease afforded by hospital isolation since the reduction took place in large part before hospital isolation became at all general, and is shared in by districts in which it is not practised. It is to be ascribed rather to scarlet fever being now a less severe disease, less often fatal to those attacked by it than it was in former years. A similar diminution has occurred in other countries also.

It has been suggested that the milder character which scarlet fever exhibits at the present day may have been brought about indirectly by hospital isolation, through a process akin to " natural selection "—the severer cases being removed to hospital, the disease would be propagated chiefly by the milder cases, which would tend to breed true. Thus Dr D. S. Davies says :

" The favourable alteration in type is probably in large part a result, not of general 'sanitary' improvement, but of the development of that part of public health work which secures removal and care in hospital for those patients who, if kept at home amongst large families in small houses, would by accumulation of infection tend to septic and fatal forms of the disease. It is in this, I believe, that much of the value of a judicious use of isolation hospitals consists ; for in large cities it is not to be expected that hospital isolation can succeed in blotting out a disease which is perennially kept going by personal infection through undiscovered cases.

" The view may be advanced, too, that in comparison with races that have not been subjected to selection by the constant presence of the scarlet fever organism in the environment, we have acquired, as a race, a very high resisting power, short of complete immunity, but so marked that the mortality caused by individuals succumbing in the process of acquiring immunity will be so small that it does not materially affect the race." (*Bristol Annual Report,* 1910.)

It is known however that the type of scarlet fever has in the past varied greatly in severity at different epochs or in different places ; at one time or place passing through a mild, at another through a severe and dangerous phase; and these variations have appeared to be independent of sanitary circumstances, preventive measures, or hereditary racial immunity. Thus Hirsch says:

"A conspicuous peculiarity of scarlet fever is the *variation in the intensity of the disease*, as seen in the degree of mortality, which in some epidemics is almost nil, or from 3 to 5 per cent. of the sick and in others 30 per cent. or more. This varying degree of severity in the disease is shown moreover not only in the successive outbreaks following close upon one another at a given place, but also in the series of epidemics distributed over longer periods of time; it comes out, too, in an equally striking way on comparing the intensity of the disease in the contemporaneous outbreaks of localities adjoining, or even throughout a wide area." He quotes the remarks of Graves, who says that in Dublin scarlet fever committed great ravages in 1801—2; in 1803—4 it changed its character, and though epidemics recurred frequently during the next 27 years, yet the disease was always in the simple or mild form. The diminished mortality was ascribed by many to the judicious employment of an antiphlogistic treatment by the Dublin physicians, but a severe epidemic in 1834—5 completely refuted this reasoning.

The prevalence of scarlet fever has clearly not declined in the same proportion as the mortality, but figures of prevalence can only be given from the dates when compulsory notification came into force[1], and then only for certain places where records have been kept. Moreover, in the earlier years notification, especially of the milder cases not attended by medical practitioners, was probably far from complete. The following table gives for London the scarlet fever notification and death-rates per 1000 population, the case-mortality per 100 cases, the percentage of cases removed to hospital and the case-mortality among cases so removed.

---

[1] Notification of infectious diseases to the Medical Officer of Health was made compulsory in various towns under local Acts of Parliament passed between 1876 and 1889. The Infectious Diseases (Notification) Act, 1889, put it in the power of any sanitary authority to adopt compulsory notification, and under an Act in 1899 it became in force in every district in England and Wales.

Scarlet Fever in London.

Period	Notification rate per 1000 living	Death-rate	Case-mortality per cent.	Percentage removed to hospital	Case-mortality in hospital
5 years, 1890–4	5·1	·24	4·9	48·4	6·8
,, 1895–9	4·6	·16	3·4	67·1	4·1
,, 1900–4	3·4	·10	2·9	80·5	3·3
,, 1905–9	4·6	·12	2·5	89·5	2·8
,, 1910–4	3·8	·05	1·5	86·4	1·7
,, 1915–9	2·4	·04	1·5	87·5	1·8
1 year, 1920	5·0	·05	0·9	91·6	1·1

It will be observed that while the percentage of cases removed to hospital has much increased the death-rate from scarlet fever has greatly diminished, the diminution being partly accounted for by a lessened number of cases, and partly by a lessened fatality of the cases that occurred. There has been, too, a marked decrease in the case mortality rate.

A similar experience is recorded at Nottingham, where scarlet fever became compulsorily notifiable in 1882, though notification was probably at first incomplete. 1882 was the last year of a formidable epidemic of scarlet fever, which had lasted since 1879 and had caused 947 deaths in the four years. This severe epidemic was followed, as is often the case, by a period of comparative quiescence, which lasted till 1888. Epidemics occurred in 1889, 1892—5, 1899—1900, 1903—4 and 1909. Hospital isolation commenced in 1885, but the number of cases removed was at first small. The proportion increased until in 1895—7 about 90 per cent. were removed. A change of policy then took place, and the medical officer of health was instructed not to remove cases from households where there were means of isolation at home, and the proportion removed fell to about one half the number notified. The following table shows the scarlet

Scarlet Fever in Nottingham.

Period	Notification rate	Death-rate	Case-mortality	Percentage removed to hospital	Average cases per household
3 years, 1882–4	3·1	·64	17·1	nil	1·16
5 years, 1885–9	2·8	·11	4·4	38	1·3
,, 1890–4	5·3	·21	4·0	81	1·24
,, 1895–9	5·1	·17	4·0	77	1·3
,, 1900–4	5·1	·13	2·4	44	1·2
,, 1905–9	2·6	·05	1·9	58	1·2
1910	2·6	·06	2·0	60	1·3
1911	1·88	·03	1·8	55	1·6

28 UTILITY OF ISOLATION HOSPITALS

fever notification and death-rates in successive periods, the case-mortality per 100 cases, the percentage of notified cases removed to hospital, and the average number of cases per household invaded.

At a discussion on Isolation Hospitals at the annual meeting of the British Medical Association at Leicester in 1905, the opinion of medical officers of health of combined areas containing rural districts and small towns, some with and others without hospital accommodation, was not favourable to the utility of hospital isolation of scarlet fever other than in exceptional cases. Dr George Wilson, medical officer of health for Mid-Warwickshire, submitted the following statistics[1]:

Mid-Warwickshire combined district. Scarlet Fever.

Periods	Aggregate districts	Mean population	Cases notified in periods	Annual attack-rate per 1000 population	Cases admitted to hospital	Percentage of admissions to cases notified	Deaths	Average annual death-rate per 1000 population	Fatality-rate per cent. of cases notified
10 years, 1892–1901	With hospitals	66,992	2868	4·28	2076	72	39	·058	1·36
	Without hospitals	52,086	1330	2·55	—	—	34	·065	2·72
3 years, 1902–4	With hospitals	82,020	1222	4·96	803	65	23	·093	1·88
	Without hospitals	57,610	831	4·80	—	—	14	·081	1·68

Dr Wilson considered that these figures showed that hospital isolation, after long years of trial, had failed to control either the incidence or the fatality-rate of scarlet fever, and that there were no grounds for assuming that it had contributed to the much milder type of the disease. He considered, too, that in mixing up mild cases with severe ones the symptoms of the former often became aggravated, and that slight cases have a better chance of recovery in their own homes; also that the risk of infection spreading in the household, however poorly circumstanced, is not nearly so great as is generally believed, more than half of the cases in the districts without hospitals being single ones in the household. But he still thought that hospitals are of use for

[1] Dr Wilson's two Tables are here condensed into one.

the reception of exceptional cases—cases for instance which crop up in connection with certain workshops, milk-shops, or dairies, or in lodging houses, or amongst servants, or severe cases which cannot be nursed at home. Severe cases should be treated in single-bed or small wards.

Similar views were expressed by Dr O'Connor, medical officer of health for the Leicestershire and Rutland Combined Districts, who submitted the following table showing the incidence of scarlet fever during the nine years 1896—1904, in a rural district in which the parishes could be divided into two groups, each of five parishes, according to the amount of hospital isolation practised, in one group from 80 to 54 per cent. of the notified cases being removed to hospital and in the other group only from 21 per cent. down to nil.

Blaby Rural District. Scarlet Fever. 1896—1904.

Groups of parishes	Population 1901	Notified cases	Removed to hospital	Percentage removed	Attack-rate per 1000 pop.
I. Hospital isolating	6,662	372	245	66	6·2
II. Home isolating	7,060	182	26	14	2·8

He attributed the inefficiency of hospital isolation as a preventive measure to the prevalence of transient atypical unnotified cases, which were the real diffusers of infection. In approximately three-fourths of initial cases in households there is not the semblance of any direct exposure to a notified case; the disease has been derived from an unascertained source; and the patients maintained in hospital are not those who most commonly spread the disease, but are those who would in any case be kept under observation and more or less effectually isolated, at least from other houses. The greater prevalence of scarlet fever in the villages which had most regularly resorted to hospital isolation he attributed to "infecting cases" in which the virulence of the infection had been enhanced by the aggregation of patients in hospital pavilions, and which gave rise to "return cases" on their discharge.

A difficulty in applying statistical tests to the question of the utility of hospital isolation in scarlet fever arises from the circumstance that the disease, like others principally affecting

children, tends in a given locality to recur in epidemic form at
intervals of several years; so that it is necessary to take for
purposes of comparison terms of years sufficiently long to include
both epidemic and inter-epidemic periods; and such a term of
years allows time, not only for a natural variation in the type of
the disease, but also for changes in the social circumstances and
age-constitution of the inhabitants which may materially affect
its incidence. And if instead of comparing the behaviour of the
disease in the same locality at different periods of time, we
institute comparison between its behaviour during the same
period in different localities varying in their extent of hospital
use, we are met with similar difficulties.

Thus, to take a case given by Dr Kaye, the following figures
had been given by Dr Millard of scarlet fever in the ten years
1890—99, in the two towns of Warrington and Preston, these
being the most effective examples in his table of "isolating"
and "non-isolating" towns.

Towns	Population (estimated)	Percentage isolated	Attack-rate	Case-mortality	Death-rate
Warrington	57,200	77	4·2	10·0	0·42
Preston	111,930	—	2·3	7·1	0·16

These figures at first sight tell strongly against hospital isolation of scarlet fever, but Dr Kaye points out that the two towns
differ greatly in regard to density, age and sex distribution, and
occupation of the inhabitants, housing accommodation, and other
matters liable to affect the incidence of scarlet fever, as shown in
the following table:

	Warrington	Preston
Number of persons per house, 1901	5·5	4·8
Persons per acre	26·7	26·3
Percentage of houses with one or two rooms only... ...	8·8	3·2
Percentage of persons living in them	5·8	1·9
Proportion per 1000 of children under 10	270	239
Mean birth-rate	36·3	33·2
School accommodation, number of seats per 100 scholars on register	107	150

He also points out that the population of Preston was shown
by the census of 1901 to have been overestimated; that under
the local Act in force in Preston till 1899, only the first case of
infectious disease in a house was notifiable; and that by taking

different periods the relative position of the two towns as regards scarlet fever incidence could be inverted. When complete notification in Preston had come into operation under the general Act of 1899 the figures of scarlet fever incidence in the next two years were:

Year	Attack-rate	Case-mortality	Death-rate
1900	4·4	6·4	0·284
1901	15·4	4·9	0·761

It is not possible to base an argument for or against the utility of hospital treatment upon a comparison of the case-mortality among cases in hospital with that of cases treated at home, for the reason that the comparative mortality of hospital-treated and home-treated cases depends largely on the initial severity of the cases as influencing removal. If hospital treatment is reserved for the more severe cases or those which have been exposed to privations and other unfavourable conditions the mortality must be expected to be greater among such cases than among the mild and well-cared-for cases which are left at home, quite irrespective of any supposed injurious hospital influence or of any ill effect of the journey. If, on the other hand, owing to the severity of the disease, the length of journey or other cause, the worst cases are not attempted to be removed, or die before removal can be effected, their inclusion among the home-treated will raise the case-mortality of this class as compared with the hospital-treated, irrespective of any benefit from hospital treatment[1].

The reasons why the practice of hospital isolation of scarlet fever, even where carried out on so large a scale as in London, has not produced a greater or more obvious diminution in the number of cases of the disease have been already mentioned. They are:

1. The occurrence during the present mild phase of scarlet

---

[1] A curious instance of how the death-rate in hospitals may be affected by extraneous circumstances is given in Bristowe and Holmes's report. At a certain hospital it was noticed that the death-rate in the wards on the ground floor was always higher than in those on the upper floor, and various explanations were offered, until it was found that the hospital porter sent patients who could walk upstairs—and who were therefore generally not seriously ill—into the upper wards, while those who had to be carried— presumably the graver cases—were taken into the ground floor wards.

fever of numerous mild or unrecognised cases, which frequently form a source of infection, at school and elsewhere. There may also perhaps be " carriers " who are capable of conveying infection without having been themselves definitely ill. So frequent are these unrecognised sources of infection, that in a large proportion of the notified cases of scarlet fever no obvious connection with any previous recognised case can be ascertained.

When however, on inquiry, such mild cases are detected they are often notified, and their inclusion helps, probably to a greater extent now than in former years, both to raise the apparent prevalence and to lower the case-mortality of the disease. Thus, also, as the result of the shifting of the point of view from the relief of the individual sufferer to the protection of the public health, the number of scarlet fever patients in hospital is augmented by the admission of slight cases, the removal of which to hospital is regarded as necessary only in order to prevent the spread of infection.

The increased opportunities for propagation of infection afforded by the greater aggregation of population at the present day have been already mentioned.

2. A frequent reason for the failure of removal to hospital of the initial case to prevent the occurrence of secondary cases is that notification and removal of the first patient often do not take place until after other members of the household have already contracted infection—scarlet fever, contrary to a former belief, being infectious from the very commencement of the symptoms. Although scarlet fever commonly commences somewhat suddenly, notification is rarely received by the medical officer of health until the second day[1], and often not till later ; and it may often not be possible for removal to be carried out on the same day on which notification is received. Hence there is usually a period of two or three days before removal during

---

[1] The medical officer of health for Woolwich in 1908 in investigating 88 cases of scarlet fever and 66 cases of diphtheria found that the intervals between the onset of illness and calling in the doctor were as follows :

	Under 1 day	2 days	3 days	4 days	5 days	6 days	8 days	10 days	11 days	13 days	15 days	16 days	18 days
Scarlet fever	10	29	24	9	1	—	—	2	1	1	1	2	1
Diphtheria	25	22	12	2	2	1	1	—	1	—	—	—	—

which the other susceptible members of the household are exposed to infection, and it is during this period that the majority of the secondary cases contract the disease.

Thus Dr Waddy of Sheffield (*British Medical Journal*, Sept. 16, 1905) said,

"Two-thirds of the total recurrence in each group of houses (viz. 690 from which scarlet fever patients were taken to hospital and 878 in which they were treated at home) took place early—that is, within 12 days of the onset of illness. Indeed in the hospital group two-thirds of the total recurrence was accounted for by cases which became ill not later than seven days after the removal of the primary case, and which might therefore be reasonably regarded as having become infected before the primary case was removed."

Secondary cases occurred in 25 per cent. of the hospital group and in only 17 per cent. of the home-treated group, but the houses from which patients go to hospital are just those which present greater possibilities of recurrence.

Similarly Dr Williamson, medical officer of health for the Epsom and Dorking Combined District, in a report in 1908, in comparing the occurrences of secondary cases in houses from which patients had been removed to hospital with that in houses in which they had been treated at home, says " Sixty per cent. of the secondary cases of scarlet fever were already infected before notification or removal of the first case ; from the end of the first week until the end of the 6th week the effect of removal (*i.e.* in preventing the occurrence of secondary cases in the households invaded) is evident ; it continues to a slight extent for the next four weeks, but is then considerably discounted by the high proportion of cases following on the return of the patient from hospital."

3. A third reason for the non-success of hospital isolation of scarlet fever cases is the liability to the occurrence of so-called "return cases," *i.e.* cases following the return home of a convalescent patient discharged from an isolation hospital. The infectious condition in a scarlet fever patient is of long, though variable, duration ; it may persist for some time after apparent recovery and may apparently revive after it has ceased on the occurrence of a sequela such as nasal catarrh. The contagium was formerly, and is still popularly, supposed to have its seat in the desquamation from the skin, but is now believed rather to reside in secretions from the mucous membranes of

the nose, throat and ears, possibly also in the urine; but the patient may apparently, in some cases, continue capable of conveying infection even when no pathological condition can be discovered. Similar "carriers" occur in diphtheria and enteric fever; but in these diseases the persistence of the infective organism can be verified by bacteriological methods, and in scarlet fever no such methods unfortunately are at present available. The liability to give rise to "return cases" is not confined to cases which have been treated in hospital, but it is commonly believed to be greater in them than in home-treated cases; and it is a constant source of anxiety to hospital managers, having often involved them in discredit, and sometimes in an action for damages in which the plaintiff obtained compensation[1].

4. The results of hospital isolation as compared with home treatment are made to appear the less favourable, by reason of the circumstance that the cases removed to hospital are in large measure selected for removal, because there are at their homes conditions—such as scant space or the presence of many susceptible inmates—which would favour the spread of infection, whereas the home-treated cases are mostly among persons better off, living in roomy houses, and with few other susceptible members in the family. When the comparison between hospital and home isolation is made, not between the percentages of released convalescents whom subsequent events prove to be infective, but between the percentages of susceptible persons in the family who are attacked after the lapse of a week (to allow for the incubation period) from the beginning of isolation of the first case, the results are much more favourable to hospital isolation.

The following figures are given by Dr Malet, M.O.H. for Wolverhampton, of the recurrence of scarlet fever after removal to hospital, and after home isolation respectively in the 13 years 1894—1906.

---

[1] In Keegan *v.* the Mayor and Corporation of Birmingham, £50 damages were obtained in the Birmingham County Court in respect of the Corporation and their officers discharging from the City Hospital a child which had not fully recovered from scarlet fever, thereby causing another child to contract the disease, in consequence whereof it died (*Public Health*, April, 1896). Similar actions however failed in the cases of Evans *v.* Mayor, etc. of Liverpool (*Public Health*, July, 1905), Jameson *v.* the Metropolitan Asylums Board, 1896, and Wright *v.* Metropolitan Asylums Board, 1904.

	Hospital isolation	Home isolation
Total houses invaded	2904	376
Cases recurred in	295	129
Number of children after primary cases	7766	721
Number of these attacked	372 or 4·8 per cent.	179 or 24·8 per cent.
Number of secondary attacks possibly due to failure of isolation	183 or 2·4 per cent.	120 or 16·6 per cent.
Number of children escaping	7394 or 95·2 per cent.	542 or 75·2 per cent.

The cases treated at home lived in roomy houses where isolation was possible.

Dr M. B. Arnold on an investigation of 2192 primary cases of scarlet fever, of which 1529 were treated in hospital and 663 were treated at home, came to the following conclusions:

1. In Manchester the great majority of the cases of scarlet fever treated at home are in houses with less than one inhabitant per room. A considerable majority of the houses from which patients are removed to hospital have one or more inhabitants per room.

2. The average number of susceptible persons per house is twice as high in the homes of the hospital cases as in the homes of the other group.

3. The difference between the percentage of susceptible persons infected in the two groups during isolation (counting only cases occurring after the 7th day) is so great that it is evident there is a great leakage of infection during home isolation.

4. When return cases[1] and recovery cases are considered with the incidental cases there is, in spite of the worse home conditions, a big gain remaining in the hospital group, the percentage of susceptible persons infected being less than half that in the group of home cases, and the actual number of cases credited to each group of 100 primary invasion cases is less

In this paper "return cases" are any occurring in the home of the patient after his return from hospital without limit of time. "Recovery cases" are cases similarly occurring after the release from isolation of a home-treated case. "Incidental cases" are cases occurring not less than 7 days after the beginning of isolation of the primary invasion cases, and before their return from hospital or release from isolation. "Primary invasion cases" include the first case and all subsequent cases occurring within 7 days of the isolation of the first or any subsequent case. "Susceptible persons" are all of the family said not to have had scarlet fever, and under 16 years old, or who being over 16 have actually contracted the disease.

than that in the home group in spite of the great difference in
the chance for infection offered. If home and hospital isolation
were adopted in a large series of similar households, the gain
demonstrated in hospital isolation would presumably be much
greater.

5. If it is allowed that a small percentage of all scarlet
fever patients remain unrecognisably infectious for longer periods
than the usual time of isolation, then the conditions to which
the hospital cases return are, in comparison with the home
treated cases, so favourable for the production of further infection, that it is probably unnecessary to seek any other explanation
of the known great excess in the percentage of return cases over
recovery cases.

To review the whole question of the advisability of the
hospital treatment of scarlet fever : there are instances in which
the patient has not the proper lodging and accommodation required for his own well-being, nor for the prevention of grave
risk of spread to other persons in the same building, *e.g.* at
a common lodging house, or in crowded houses of people of the
poorer class. There are severe or complicated cases in which
the patient requires the treatment and nursing which he can
obtain at a hospital better than in his own home. Cases also
occur under circumstances in which to allow the patient to
remain at home would involve grave risk or alarm to the general
public, as for instance at a dairy, or at a post office or other
frequented place of business ; or where his remaining might
involve serious pecuniary loss, as at an hotel or a boarding
school. In such exceptional cases the propriety of removing
the patient to a suitable hospital will hardly be disputed ; they
must be expected to occur from time to time in any populous
district, and a local authority which has not provided hospital
accommodation suitable and sufficient to meet them, must be
regarded as having failed in discharging an obvious public
duty. On the other hand it is doubtful whether the removal to
hospital, as a routine practice, of every scarlet fever patient
willing to go, is advisable on grounds of health, or is worth the
expenditure which it involves. If scarlet fever were to revert to

the severe type of former years it might be otherwise ; but in its present mild phase too many cases are passed over to render the isolation of those which are recognised of much avail in checking the spread of the disease ; and mild cases do well under home treatment, and avoid certain dangers which they might incur by being aggregated with other patients in hospital. This especially applies in time of an epidemic, when the attempt to get every patient into hospital has before now led to serious over-crowding of the wards to the detriment of the patients and of the health of the nurses. It is also inadvisable that a local authority should reserve its hospital for cases of scarlet fever, to the exclusion of more serious diseases, such as enteric fever or diphtheria[1].

In some districts it has been the practice to attempt to remove to hospital as large a proportion of scarlet fever cases as possible ; in others no hospital accommodation is available, or such as there is is used for scarlet fever only in rare and exceptional cases. But between these two extremes lie a large number of instances in which the proportion of cases, whether greater or less, in which removal may be deemed expedient is governed by local conditions. In districts in which many of the inhabitants get their living by occupations which would be interfered with by the presence of infectious disease in their houses, as by letting lodgings at a health resort, by keeping boarding schools, or by laundry or other home work, the demand for removal of scarlet fever cases to hospital will be greater than in, say, an agricultural or mining district. There is, therefore, room for legitimate differences of opinion among local authorities and their advisers as to the extent to which it is advisable to resort to hospital isolation of scarlet fever cases.

[1] The following resolution proposed by Dr Millard at a meeting of the Midland Branch of the Society of Medical Officers of Health may be quoted as embodying the views of an able critic of hospital isolation (*Public Health*, May, 1902):

"That whilst the provision of hospital isolation for persons suffering from scarlet fever is a very great convenience to the public, it is doubtful, from the point of view of controlling the disease, whether the results achieved by the wholesale removal of cases to hospital are commensurate with the heavy cost entailed. It is possible that results equally satisfactory would be obtained by the removal to hospital of the more urgent cases only.

" Also in no case is the wholesale removal to hospital of scarlet fever cases to be recommended if it involves overcrowding of the available hospital accommodation."

In the case of diphtheria and enteric fever, the two other diseases at the present time most commonly admitted into isolation hospitals, the advantages of hospital treatment are less open to question, although objections similar to those raised to the hospital isolation of scarlet fever, have sometimes been raised to that of diphtheria. It is true that some of the cases now included as diphtheria are mild and untypical, and are only recognised as diphtheritic on bacteriological examination, but "clinical" diphtheria is a serious disease, requiring skilled nursing and in some cases operation; and it is liable to be followed by local paralyses and sometimes by sudden death from heart failure. Enteric fever is also a formidable disease, and is very liable to spread under the conditions of housing and nursing met with in households of the poorer class; it is now recognised to be much more readily communicable from person to person than was formerly supposed, and nurses frequently contract it[1]. It is not now so often received into general hospitals as formerly; and it is commonly to the patient's advantage that he should go into an isolation hospital if he is able to bear the journey.

All isolation hospitals are liable to receive a number of cases which turn out not to be of the disease which had been diagnosed before they were sent in. Mistakes of this kind are not always avoidable, for it often happens that a patient develops feverishness or other symptoms resembling the beginning of some infectious disease, under circumstances in which it is important for his own sake, or for the safety of others, that he should be removed at once, since to wait until the diagnosis had been confirmed would involve a delay which might permit the spread of infection, or the patient might then be too ill to bear removal. Such erroneous diagnoses occurred in 10·6 per cent. of all the admissions into the fever hospitals of the Metropolitan Asylums Board in 1911, the percentage on the total scarlet fever cases being 8·7, on the diphtheria cases, 12·7, and on the enteric fever cases 34·2. Among the small-pox cases, which are verified

---

[1] In the Fever hospitals of the Metropolitan Asylums Board in 1911 the mortality among scarlet fever cases was 1·94 per cent., diphtheria 8·9, "bacteriological diphtheria" 2·02, enteric fever 14·3, measles 13·89, and whooping-cough 13·24.

by a medical officer at the London wharves before being sent to hospital, the percentage of mistakes in diagnosis was found to be 22·0. Thus the proportion of mistakes is greater in the more formidable and dangerous diseases, viz. in those which call especially for early removal. The diseases most frequently mistaken for scarlet fever were rubella (German measles), tonsillitis, and erythema ; for diphtheria, tonsillitis, and for enteric fever, influenza, tuberculosis and pneumonia, while in respect of each disease there were a number of cases sent to hospital in which no obvious illness could be found on examination.

Besides this a patient sent in with one disease may also be incubating a second infectious disease, and this is especially liable to happen where the second disease is one with a long incubation period, as measles, whooping-cough, rubella, chicken-pox, or mumps. Hence these diseases, though not ordinarily admissible into isolation hospitals, are liable to be introduced from time to time, especially into children's wards, where they are apt to spread among the patients, and in the absence of special means of isolation may give rise to troublesome outbreaks, though in the case of the three last named there is no appreciable mortality. For these reasons it happens that a certain number of cases of these non-notifiable or minor infectious diseases are often treated in isolation hospitals.

Apart, however, from such casual introductions measles and whooping-cough have since 1910 been received into the Metropolitan Asylum Board's fever hospitals, with a view of saving life in severe cases occurring in households of the poorer class, rather than with a view of controlling infection. The long incubation period of these diseases, their special incidence on very young children, and their early infectiousness before the characteristic rash or cough has appeared, render any attempt to check the spread of infection by hospital isolation far from hopeful. On this point, in a report to the Metropolitan Asylums Board in 1910, Dr H. E. Cuff says :

" Measles and whooping-cough are so highly infectious in their early stages, before a diagnosis as a rule is made, that isolation is much less likely to affect their prevalence than it is in the case of the notifiable diseases. For this reason very few authorities make any provision for their treatment. This, it seems to me, is looking at the question from too narrow a point of view. That isolation will have but little influence on the prevalence of measles and whooping-cough seems certain, but is the possibility of saving life and of promoting a complete instead of a partial restoration to health not to be taken into consideration?" Both measles and whooping-cough are attended with complications and sequelæ which if left uncured may shorten life or seriously impair the future usefulness of the individual. More persons attribute their deafness to measles than to scarlet fever and there is no doubt that a considerable proportion of deaf mutes owe their disability to the former disease. Defective vision and even blindness, usually one-sided, may be left after measles. These serious affections of sight and hearing are especially likely to occur in badly nourished children living in unhealthy surroundings." He says "the foregoing considerations would appear to establish a case for the hospital treatment of selected cases of measles and whooping-cough, not because they are infectious diseases, but because children suffering from them stand in urgent need of good air, good food and good nursing; consequently they would be admitted for curative rather than for preventive reasons." He points out that Dr Wilson in a paper on the prevalence and mortality of measles in Aberdeen during the 20 years that compulsory notification was in force there, showed that the death-rate (? case-mortality) among children who lived in one-roomed houses was 7 to 8 times greater than among those who lived in houses containing four or five rooms. Similar figures had shown the effect of poverty and overcrowding upon the death-rate of whooping-cough. It is true that the mortality of measles is greater among hospital treated cases than in private practice, the reason being that the former are selected for admission on account of the poverty of their surroundings and would therefore include a number of weakly ill-nourished babies; while the home-treated cases would probably include many of German measles, a disease which never proves fatal.

Dr Ker, of the City Hospital, Edinburgh, is confident that a large number of the children suffering from measles, who pass through the wards of the hospital, would certainly have died if they had been left at home.

From a report made by Dr Chalmers, M.O.H., of Glasgow, in 1910, it appears that measles and whooping-cough have been treated in hospital at that city since 1891, the proportion of cases admitted to hospital to the total number registered being about 11 per cent. of the cases of measles and 25 per cent. of those of whooping-cough. He shows that during that period there had been a great decline (about 35 per cent.) in the death-rate from whooping-cough, and a distinct though smaller decline (13 per cent.) in the death-rate from measles in the city. The death-rate from both measles and whooping-cough had fallen more rapidly in Glasgow than in the rest of Scotland.

A circumstance which may facilitate the treatment of selected cases of measles and whooping-cough in isolation hospitals is that the greatest prevalence of these diseases is in the first half of the year while the greatest prevalence of scarlet fever, diphtheria and enteric fever is in the latter half of the year. Accommodation for the former would therefore be likely to be most required at a time when the wards were comparatively empty.

In the hospitals of the Metropolitan Asylums Board during 1911, the case-mortality among measles patients was 13·5 per cent. and among those with whooping-cough 12·2 per cent. ; these high rates are ascribed to only the most urgent and necessitous cases being admitted. Of the cases that recovered, the average length of stay in hospital was, measles 41 days, among those treated throughout in town hospitals, and 59·4 days among those transferred to convalescent hospitals ; whooping-cough 78·5 days and 82·8 days, under similar conditions respectively.

Puerperal fever, under which term are included the septic affections which may follow child-birth, is occasionally admitted into isolation hospitals, sometimes—as at the Monsall Hospital, Manchester, and Fazakerly Hospital, Liverpool—with the special object of carrying out operative measures.

Erysipelas, and in recent years, cerebro-spinal fever and acute anterior poliomyelitis, are occasionally treated in isolation hospitals, usually in the patient's own interest, rather than with a view to his isolation.

Typhus is a disease now rarely met with in this country, except in a few northern towns. When it occurs its victims are persons of the poorest class living in squalid and overcrowded dwellings, and hence their removal to hospital is always necessary[1].

Cholera in the epidemics of former years, and so lately as the threatened outbreak of 1892, led frequently to the provision of temporary hospital accommodation, especially at seaports. The fact that cholera patients bear removal badly, and, as it is considered, cannot safely be carried distances greater than a mile, renders it necessary that the accommodation provided should be close to the spot where the disease is likely to occur, and hence such accommodation has usually taken the form of sheds, huts, or tents, or the fitting up of an existing building.

Small-pox is the disease which perhaps exemplifies best the advantage of isolation in a suitable hospital in preventing the spread of infection[2]. The dread entertained of the disease renders it generally easy to obtain consent to early removal; the "contacts" and nurses can be rendered immune by vaccination, and there appears to be in small-pox no liability to the prolonged persistence or recurrence of infectiveness after apparent

[1] The recent discovery that typhus and relapsing fever are transmitted by the bites of insect parasites would, if these diseases should again become established in this country, involve a reconsideration in this new light of the old problems referred to in the first chapter. It is possible also that the virus of typhus may have suffered an attenuation similar to that which the contagia of scarlet fever and small-pox seem to have undergone. When typhus occurs nowadays it may get a certain footing before its nature is discovered, owing to the unfamiliarity of the present generation of medical practitioners with the disease; but when once detected it is usually soon stamped out, and does not exhibit the virulence and capacity for extensive spread which made it so dreaded fifty years ago.

[2] Dr D. S. Davies says: "The conception which early followed the discovery of the specific pathogenic bacteria, that they entered, permeated, and then passed out of the body like an orderly army, leaving no stragglers, is found in many cases to be far from the truth. Had it been true the efficacy of isolation hospitals would have been complete, and the control of infectious fevers would have proved an almost crudely simple matter. As we shall see later it possibly is true with regard to one disease, small-pox, so that in certain respects this is one of the diseases most amenable to control in spite of its intense infectivity."

recovery, which so often causes difficulty with scarlet fever and diphtheria. At the present time, when small-pox spreads it is usually because the nature of the first cases has not been recognised at a sufficiently early stage.

Owing, however, to the highly diffusible nature of the contagion of small-pox, it cannot safely be treated in the same hospital with other diseases, even in a detached building, and the need for separate small-pox hospitals was early recognised. They must not be near populous localities (see Chapter IX).

Since the discovery of the bacillus tuberculosis by Koch in 1882, the infectious nature of "open" cases—*i.e.* cases with external discharges—of tuberculosis has come to be generally admitted and public opinion has been brought to see the importance of taking all practicable action to hasten the diminution of the large mortality and disability caused by tuberculous diseases, especially phthisis.

During the last decade of the nineteenth century and the first decade of the present, it had become the practice in some areas to use isolation hospitals at times, when their beds would otherwise be unoccupied, for cases of pulmonary tuberculosis. The treatment of tuberculous patients at these hospitals was considerably extended by the passing of the National Insurance Act, 1912. Up to that time relatively few local authorities had undertaken the treatment of tuberculosis, and the number of beds available in institutions specially provided for this class of case throughout the country was quite inadequate to meet the needs of the County and County Borough Councils and the Insurance Committees. To assist in meeting this demand local authorities in some areas rearranged the working of their isolation hospitals, as for example, by treating cases of enteric fever in observation blocks instead of in pavilions provided originally for that disease. By these means it was found possible to devote single pavilions at various hospitals to the treatment of tuberculosis. Such arrangements were approved by the late Local Government Board, subject to the condition that the pavilion should revert temporarily to the treatment of acute infectious disease if necessary. Similarly certain small-pox hospitals were used, and continue to be so used, for accommodating tuberculous patients. In these instances arrangements have to be made by the hospital authority for the treatment of sporadic cases of small-pox occurring in their area in the small-pox hospitals belonging to other authorities. This arrangement obviates the need for evacuating tuberculous patients from the hospital except in the event of an outbreak threatening to assume epidemic proportions. The small-pox hospital and its contents must of course be thoroughly disinfected and cleansed before being used again for tuberculous cases.

The advantages to be gained by providing for the treatment of tuberculous patients at isolation hospitals, furthermore led some authorities to erect new pavilions for tuberculous cases in the grounds of, or adjacent to, existing isolation hospitals. Generally speaking isolation hospitals are not suitably situated or well adapted for the treatment of true sanatorium cases, that is to say, those in which there is a prospect of arrest of the disease and the restoration, for a time at least, of full working capacity. Pavilions at isolation hospitals are, however, very suitable for the following purposes :

(1) Observation of persons suspected to be suffering from tuberculosis. It is desirable that provision for this purpose should be conveniently situated for the tuberculosis officer, and this can sometimes be secured by making the necessary provision at an isolation hospital. It is important that patients admitted with a view to diagnosis should have sleeping accommodation separate from that used by patients who are definitely tuberculous.

(2) Observation of definite cases of tuberculosis with a view to ascertaining whether they are likely to be benefitted by sanatorium treatment.

(3) Short period treatment of patients in whose cases there is no prospect of securing the arrest of the disease, with a view of restoring health temporarily and educating these persons in habits of living which may conduce not only to their own benefit but to the safety of other people with whom they may live after leaving the hospital. Patients when in a somewhat advanced stage of pulmonary tuberculosis are often found to benefit markedly by the rest, attention, good food and fresh air which they get in a well appointed hospital : a comparatively short stay which may have to be repeated several times, may temporarily restore working

capacity; or at least give the patient the best chance of securing improved health.

(4) Treatment of patients whose disease is in an advanced stage, with a view of ameliorating the condition of the sufferers as far as possible and preventing the spread of infection in their homes (see also chapter on Sanatoria for Tuberculosis, p. 220).

BIBLIOGRAPHY

6th Report of Medical Officer of Privy Council. 1863. With Report by Bristowe and Holmes on the Hospitals of the United Kingdom.

Annual Reports of Registrar General.

Seaton, E. C. Infectious Diseases and their Preventive Treatment. 1910.

Davies, D. S. Annual Report for Bristol. 1910.

—— Diphtheria and Small Pox, an epidemiological contrast. Public Health, March, 1909.

Hirsch. Handbook of Geographical and Historical Pathology. Sydenham Society's Translation. 1883.

Annual Reports of Metropolitan Asylums Board.

Annual Reports of Medical Officer of Health for Nottingham.

Wilson, J. T. A contribution to the natural history of Scarlet Fever. Public Health, Feb., 1897.

Cameron, R. W. D. M. Concerning the utility of Isolation Hospitals. Public Health, April, 1897.

British Medical Journal. Sept. 10, 1905. Containing papers by Drs George Wilson, J. E. O'Connor and Waddy.

Fitzsimmon, J. B. Influence of Hospital Isolation on Scarlet Fever in Hereford. Public Health, March, 1905.

Millard, C. Killick. The influence of Hospital Isolation in Scarlet Fever. Public Health, Feb., 1901.

—— The hospital treatment of Scarlet Fever; some points of uncertainty. Public Health, Feb., 1902.

Fraser, E. Mearns. Is the hospital isolation of Scarlet Fever worth while? Public Health, Jan., 1904.

Willoughby. The value of Hospitals for Scarlet Fever. Public Health, March, 1905.

Scatterty, W. Hospital Isolation. Ibid.

Wilkinson, E. Municipal Control of Zymotic Disease. Ibid.

Malet, H. Hospital and Home treatment of Scarlet Fever. Public Health, Sept., 1909.

Arnold, M. B. The relation of Housing to the isolation of Scarlet Fever and to Return cases. Trans. of Epidemiological Section, Royal Society of Medicine. March 22, 1912.

Sweeting, R. D. Report on prevalence of Scarlet Fever at Weymouth, in annual report of Medical Officer Local Government Board. 1901—2.

Gordon, A. Knyvett. On the sources of infection in Puerperal Fever. Public Health, Jan., 1906.

Cuff, H. E. Memorandum on utilization of spare accommodation at fever hospitals, in Report of Metropolitan Asylums Board. 1910.

Chalmers. Memorandum on Hospitals. Glasgow. 1910.

Bulstrode, H. T. Report to Local Government Board on Sanatoria for Consumption and certain other aspects of the Tuberculosis question. 1908. [C. 3657.]

Fremantle, F. C. The value of Isolation Hospitals. Public Health, Oct., 1906.

Kaye, J. R. Scarlet Fever; how far do statistics prove or disprove the utility of Hospital Isolation? Public Health, May, 1902.

Newsholme, A. On the notification of doubtful cases and the hospital isolation of Scarlet Fever and Diphtheria. Ibid.

—— The epidemiology of Scarlet Fever in relation to the utility of Isolation Hospitals. Transactions of Epidemiological Society. 1900—1.

Crookshank, F. G. The control of Scarlet Fever. Proceedings of Epidemiological Section, Royal Society of Medicine. Jan. 28, 1910.

Chalmers, A. K. Presidential Address on the Functions of Isolation Hospitals. Transactions Epidemiological Section of the Royal Society of Medicine for 1920.

CHAPTER III

SUBSTITUTES FOR HOSPITAL ISOLATION

IT is not necessary, or probably desirable, that every case of the ordinary infectious diseases should be removed to hospital. If the patient has proper lodging and accommodation at his home, and is able to procure suitable food, medical attendance, and good nursing, and if there are no susceptible persons to be endangered, or he can be effectually isolated from the rest of the household, except those in attendance on him, his removal to hospital is not called for on grounds of public health, though even in such cases it may be desired by the householder on grounds of convenience[1].

[1] Dr Chapin, Superintendent of Health of the City of Providence, U.S.A., says, upon a basis of 1737 cases, "It has been shown that when families with more than one susceptible child are attacked with scarlet fever, and no pretence at isolation is made, the disease spreads beyond the first case in about 55 %, involving 54·8 % of the children in these families. When isolation is fairly maintained however it spreads beyond the first case in 35·3 %, and involves 40·1 % of the children. Thus

But in households of the poorer class it is often otherwise, and even though the patient may have, in fair measure, the accommodation, food and attendance needful for his own welfare, he often has to share a room with other persons, and to be nursed by the housewife, who has to prepare the food, and perform other offices for the rest of the household ; and under these conditions there must be risk of spread of infection. Also the presence of a case of infectious disease in the house necessitates the other children being kept from school, and in the case of some occupations may interfere with the employment of the wage-earner. These difficulties are best met by the removal of the patient to an isolation hospital ; but as the authorities of the smaller urban and rural districts are frequently averse, from fear of expense or other reasons, to providing hospitals, other methods have been from time to time suggested.

Temporary places for the reception of the sick. When a serious epidemic has occurred in a place unprovided with an isolation hospital, existing buildings of various kinds and degrees of suitability, have on occasion been pressed into the service.

The objections to all such makeshift arrangements are :

1st. That they are not ready in time to receive the early cases, and indeed often not until the course of the epidemic is far advanced.

2nd. That the accommodation is often of an unsuitable kind, entailing difficulties in administration.

it will be seen that isolation as ordinarily carried out has a very considerable protective power, considerably more than the above figures would indicate, for quite a proportion of the 'secondary' cases are not really secondary but were exposed to the same contagion as the primary case, and of course could not have been protected by any isolation. It is very rare indeed that perfect isolation is attempted when sick and well are kept in the same house. Yet the somewhat imperfect attempts that are made are, I think, of undoubted value.

"It is only by the removal of the well children from the house, or the placing of the sick person in a hospital, that real isolation can in most cases be secured. The value of such removal of well children is shown by the fact that of 317 children who were at once removed only 18 or 5·6 % were attacked on their return. If these children had remained at home, doubtless half of them would have yielded to the disease." *Public Health*, Nov. 1895.

Scarlet fever does not however usually exhibit in this country at the present time so high a degree of communicability as is indicated by Dr Chapin's figures.

3rd.   That it is not of use after the epidemic is over.

In some instances a schoolroom, out of use for the time owing to the school having been closed on account of the epidemic, has been converted into a temporary hospital, requiring of course to be very thoroughly disinfected before reverting to its ordinary use.

The following are examples, taken from the Hospital Return of 1895, of some of the kinds of buildings which have in emergencies been used or proposed to be used as isolation hospitals, the descriptions being those given by the local authorities themselves[1], proper names being omitted.

" Part of disused pottery converted into a small-pox hospital, but the building is not a suitable one."

"Old disused Corporation harbour offices.   No separate accommodation for the two sexes, but a partition could be put up."

" Upper floor of a building formerly used as the borough gaol in the middle of the town.   The hospital, which is in a most unsuitable position, has never been used."

"Building formerly used for ship-building purposes."

"Five small rooms under same roof as store attached to the gas works."

" In 1887 the Sanitary Authority purchased two railway carriages and erected them on the beach near the harbour for cholera cases only."

"Formerly a weaving mill."

"A barn converted into a cottage."

"Store houses on the quay, fitted up for cholera patients arriving by sea."

" An old warehouse on river bank."

"An old granary on shore, converted into a hospital at a trivial cost.   No area of land around it."

" An old powder magazine has been purchased, but nothing has been done to prepare it for the reception of patients."

"Governor's house of the old borough gaol."

"Corrugated iron building for small-pox on disused colliery siding."

" An old glass-bottle factory, temporarily used for small-pox."

Disused workhouses in several cases.

Cottages ordinarily in use as dwellings used on emergency for isolation.   In a number of rural and small urban districts, it was said, in the Hospital Return of 1895, that the sanitary authority had hired isolated cottages or houses for use as hospitals when outbreaks of infectious disease had occurred. Sometimes the house had been given up when the outbreak

In several of the districts from which these replies were received more suitable hospital accommodation has since been provided.

was over ; in other cases, possession was still retained, but the number of cases isolated was small.

Sometimes the house was let to a tenant on condition that he turned out when it was required for use as a hospital.

At Bodmin, a three-roomed house and premises 40 (? square) yards in extent, belonging to the Urban Sanitary Authority, were kept available as a hospital. "Tenant turns out at 24 hours' notice." No cases had been admitted during the years 1888—92.

At Louth the hospital was a cottage ordinarily used as a residence by one of the U.S.A.'s labourers. When required for use as a hospital the man and his family were sent elsewhere. Nine cases of small-pox were admitted in 1888, and three of other diseases in 1890.

At Diss the hospital accommodation consisted of a double cottage leased from the churchwardens, to which extra rooms had been added. Furniture was kept in one end of the cottage, and the other was let to a tenant who would turn out if the place were required as a hospital. No case had however been admitted in the five years 1888—92, although diphtheria had been prevalent during several of those years.

A similar arrangement formerly existed at the Pest House at Huntingdon, mentioned in Chapter I, and it was in consequence rarely used.

Arrangement with householders to receive infectious cases. In a memorandum issued by the late Local Government Board in 1876, it was suggested that in a village a permanent arrangement might be made beforehand with trustworthy cottagers not having children, that they should receive and nurse in case of need patients requiring such accommodation. This suggestion has sometimes been adduced by local authorities as showing that the provision of a hospital was unnecessary, but no instance is known to the writer of this book in which it has actually been carried out. Apart from the difficulty of finding suitable people to undertake the office, cottages which would be suitable for the purpose are often scarce in country villages ; and a couple who had more house-room than they required would have no difficulty in letting rooms to lodgers.

P.

4

Hiring infected house as temporary hospital. A plan which was formerly recommended by the late Mr J. Makinson Fox, medical officer for Mid-Cheshire, was to hire for the time being from the occupier, the house in which a case of infectious disease existed, to remove the healthy inmates and put a nurse in charge, thus, it was claimed, converting the house into a " temporary place for the reception of the sick," such as the authority were empowered to provide by § 131, Public Health Act, 1875. The expenses incurred however were disallowed by the District auditors and the Local Government Board sustained the objection.

Tents. It is sometimes contended by local authorities that if the need for hospital accommodation arose they could in the course of a few hours procure and erect tents or huts. It has however to be remembered that before tents or huts erected on emergency can be available for the reception of patients a site has to be found on which permission to erect them can be obtained—not always an easy matter. The site has also to be prepared, a water supply and means of drainage provided, furniture and other necessary equipment procured, nurses engaged, and supplies arranged for ; and all these things take time and cost money.

A system of hospital tents kept in stock with the necessary equipment, and ready to be transported from place to place as occasion requires, was in operation for several years in certain Essex districts, under the care of Dr J. W. Cook, who however, stated that even in this case difficulties such as have been mentioned were met with, and recommended in preference the combination of districts for the provision of a centrally situated permanent hospital. In his annual report for 1909 on the Tendring Rural District he said :

" The isolation hospital consists of two tents, containing four beds each, for patients, and a bell-tent for two nurses, with a large van fitted up as, and used as, a kitchen, when the hospital is at work. At other times the van contains all the appurtenances of the hospital, so that it can be moved about from place to place as may be required ; but there is, and must be, considerable loss of time in getting it erected and put to work. Land has to be procured and nurses obtained, besides the erection of the tents, and then only one disease can be treated at a time. I have often regretted that we had no proper permanent hospital, but never more so than during the Scarlet Fever epidemic of last year, for, had there been a hospital ready so that the first cases could have been moved and placed under proper isolation, I feel sure the outbreak would have been stopped in a very short time, and that the cases would have been few."

In a rural district in another county a portable hospital was purchased by the District Council and was erected on a site within the district, under an agreement by which the Council were compelled to remove it at the end of six months. It was afterwards stacked in a shed. Numerous attempts to find a new site for it were made, but were always frustrated on account of opposition in the localities selected, and in the end the hospital had to be sold.

It is commonly found, with all such temporary arrangements, that the local authority are unwilling to incur the expense of bringing them into operation when the outbreak is as yet limited to one or two cases only, although this is the time when isolation would be of most service, preferring to wait and see if it becomes more serious. When the outbreak has become serious, the period of the hospital's greatest usefulness is past. The same remark applies to arrangements which involve the inconvenience of displacing a tenant.

The cost of dealing with outbreaks of infectious disease by temporary expedients is often considerable. A single case of small-pox treated at home has cost the District Council as much as £120, in another instance £63, and in another two cases cost £142.

The removal of the unaffected persons from the house in which infectious disease exists is a course which is sometimes feasible, and appears to have been formerly resorted to during outbreaks of cholera, when the patient was too ill to bear removal. An objection to this course is that the persons removed may themselves be incubating the disease, and may thus convey it to the places to which they have been removed ; they may also contract it on their return home, see footnote on p. 47.

4—2

Section 61, Public Health Acts Amendment Act, 1907, in districts where it has been put in force, enacts that where the local authority have provided a temporary shelter or house accommodation, they may, on the appearance of any infectious disease in a house, and on the certificate of the medical officer, cause any person who is not himself sick, and who consents to leave the house, or whose parent or guardian consents on his behalf, to be removed therefrom to any such temporary shelter or house accommodation. If he does not consent an order for his removal may be made by two justices. The removal is, in any case, to be effected without charge to the person removed, or his parent or guardian.

Payment of wage-earner to abstain from work. A course which has sometimes been advocated as a means of avoiding danger of infection to the public in cases where a patient suffering from an infectious disease has to be retained at home, owing to the absence of an isolation hospital, is to pay the wages of the head of the household in order that he may keep away from work. Where the wage-earner is engaged in milking, or in handling food, his continuing at work while infectious disease is in the house might, no doubt, be dangerous ; but in the case of workers in the open air the risk may be considered negligible, and even in the case of indoor workers, as in factories, it is rare for infectious disease, other than small-pox, to be contracted from a " contact " not himself ill, and any risk may be greatly diminished by attention to cleanliness of the person and clothing. Moreover, it has happened that a man who had been paid to stay away from his work has been found frequenting public-houses, or otherwise exposing himself in ways involving at least as much danger to the public as if he had been at work.

In industrial districts a chief means of spread of infectious disease from household to household (next perhaps to school attendance) is the visiting and intercourse which, through motives of sympathy, friendliness or curiosity, goes on between the infected household and neighbours. There is no legal means of forbidding the visits of neighbours to an infected person, and the keeping of the children from school, and of the elder members of the infected household from work, in no way prevents this intercourse—school-closing may perhaps even promote it ; so that unless the infection is to be allowed to run its natural course, the only way is to remove the patient to hospital.

"*Watcher-messenger*" *Method*. Another method is that thus described by Dr Spencer Low in his report to the Local Government Board in 1907 on the sanitary circumstances and administration of the Hartley Wintney Rural District :

"Isolation of sick persons is not practised ; no isolation hospital is available owing to the refusal of the District Council either to provide one themselves or to enter into arrangements with other local authorities for the purpose. The cottages of the working classes in this district as a rule barely contain sufficient accommodation for their occupants in times of health. During the course of an infectious illness in such a house the remaining inmates of the household have to run the risk of contracting the disease.

"Reliance is placed upon what is locally called the 'Watcher-messenger' system, a man being employed by the Council to spend the day in the vicinity of the infected cottage to keep people away from it and to go messages to the shops, fetch water and so on. Children in neighbouring cottages are sometimes excluded from school and on occasion these with the children of the invaded house play with the convalescent patient or patients, who are still of course infectious. Owing to the mildness of the type of scarlet fever which is now common probably little loss of life is to be anticipated from this system so long as the circumstances remain the same. In case of diphtheria, however, contacts who are unprotected by antitoxin and who are not promptly attended by a medical man when they are attacked run a grave danger. Further the fact that the mother is usually the nurse in case of enteric fever and at the same time prepares food for her family renders the inmates of the invaded household liable to become infected with that disease.

"Complaint had been made to the Board about the time of my visit of the defective isolation arrangements in force at a village where some cases of scarlatina had occurred. At one house a child was desquamating and playing in the garden with

its brothers and sisters and with children from an adjoining
house ; the mother of the patient was shortly to be confined. In
another house the patient was desquamating freely, but he had
been walking in the lane which was patrolled by the messenger,
permission to leave his premises having been given the patient
by his medical attendant, so it was said. In a third house the
patient was playing in the garden with her brothers and sisters,
some of whom showed definite signs of desquamation though
they had not been reported to have had scarlatina. The mother
had, the day before my visit, been attacked by that disease.
Beyond the fact that the messenger was useful in acting as
a servant to these cottagers by going their messages I could not
see what good purpose he was serving, or why he should be paid
by the Council. I have grave doubts whether this 'watcher-
messenger' system is worth the expenditure incurred upon it.
The messenger does not always interfere with children in adjacent cottages playing with the convalescent, and he must needs
be off duty at night and unavailable as a guard by day while
going messages."

In one case mentioned the cost of the "watcher-messenger"
was £7. 10s.

Visiting by District Nurses. It has been claimed that by
the employment of district nurses or health visitors to visit
houses in which infectious disease exists much can be done to
prevent the spread of disease to other members of the household
or to neighbours, even without removal of the patient to hospital.
The nurse could not be constantly on guard; her functions
would be to instruct the mother as to the precautions which
should be carried out in the way of isolation, disinfection and
cleanliness. The plan is said to have been at one time in
successful operation at Hastings[1]. It is most likely perhaps to
be useful in the case of diseases affecting young children, as
measles and whooping-cough, in which removal to hospital is

[1] Evidence of Mrs F. Johnstone before Royal Commission on Small-Pox and
Fever Hospitals, 1882.

This system is not mentioned in Dr Bruce Low's Report in 1894 on Diphtheria
and Small-Pox at Hastings, so it is to be presumed that it had then either been given
up, or was not considered to play an important part in the sanitary defences of the
town.

often impracticable, and in which the excess of mortality among the working class as compared with the well-to-do shows that bad home conditions and defective nursing contribute largely to the fatality. Section 67, Public Health Acts Amendment Act, where it has been put in force, enacts that

(1) "The local authority may provide nurses for attendance on patients suffering from any infectious disease in their district, who, owing to want of accommodation at the hospital or danger of infection, cannot be removed to the hospital, or in cases where removal to the hospital is likely to endanger the patient's health." (2) The local authority may charge such reasonable sums for the service of nurses provided by them as they think fit. It is, however, stipulated that (3) "Nothing in this section shall be deemed to take away or diminish the necessity of providing proper hospital accommodation for persons suffering from infectious disease."

Eucalyptus Treatment. It has been suggested that the hospital isolation of scarlet fever might be rendered unnecessary by the adoption of the treatment of inunction with eucalyptus oil originally advocated by the late Mr Brendon Curgenven and more recently revived in a modified form by Dr Robert Milne, medical officer to Dr Barnardo's Homes. During the first four days in a scarlet fever case, commencing at the earliest possible moment, pure eucalyptus oil is gently rubbed in, morning and evening, all over the body from the crown of the head to the soles of the feet. Afterwards this is repeated once a day until the tenth day of the disease. The tonsils are swabbed with 1 in 10 carbolic oil every two hours for the first twenty-four hours, rarely longer. Dr Milne says: "When this treatment is commenced early— and I emphasize the fact that early treatment is vital—secondary infection never occurs, and complications are unknown." " With this treatment carefully carried out I have no hesitation in allowing children to occupy the same room or even sleep in the same bed. The mother is free to attend to both the patient and her duties, the father is free to go to work without the slightest risk, and the children are equally free to attend school."

The experience of medical superintendents who have tried this method in hospital does not altogether bear out these statements. Thus at the Plaistow hospital during the year in which it was employed in every case of scarlet fever, Dr Biernacki stated that cross infections became commoner; a number of probationers acquired scarlet fever in the course of their duties; doubtful cases contracted scarlet fever from genuine cases in the wards and in the convalescent home; there was an increased prevalence of septic complications, particularly otitis, among the scarlet fever patients ; and the number of return cases rose above the average. Dr Milne attributed this unfavourable experience to the circumstance that in hospital practice the medical attendant was unable to apply the treatment at the earliest period of the disease, and he regarded that as of vital moment. But this explanation renders it clear that—even if the treatment can do all that is claimed for it, under the conditions of an institution such as an orphanage, where the children are continually under observation and the initial symptoms of scarlet fever, such as sore throat, vomiting, and feverishness can be at once detected— it cannot be effectually applied to scarlet fever in the general community where notification of a case is rarely, if ever, received on the first day and often not for several days after its commencement, by which time other persons have already contracted infection. Moreover the carrying out of the treatment with the prescribed frequency would be impracticable in most households without the aid of a trained nurse ; and even if the local authority were empowered to engage and pay nurses their employment on a scale sufficient to cope with a serious outbreak of scarlet fever would be very costly. There would also still be a proportion of cases in which removal to hospital was needed on account of want of accommodation or special danger to the public.

In his annual report for 1910, Dr Park, M.O.H. for Dukinfield, gives an account of 18 months' trial of the eucalyptus treatment in that borough, and reports that he is satisfied with the results. At the same time his report shows that the difficulties mentioned above have in practice been experienced. He says: " At the end of the first half-year's working the general opinion among the medical men of the district was that they could not rely on the treatment—particularly the throat treatment—being carried out effectually. To do so a capable nurse should be employed." He recommends that one should be provided by the Town Council, but this advice does not appear to have been followed by them.

Dr Park states that in 1908, before the treatment was adopted, there were 112 notified cases of scarlet fever, of which 38 were duplicate cases. In 1910 there were 52 cases notified, and in six houses duplicate cases occurred, 14 in all. In one house two and in another three cases took the disease at the same time and were notified together. In a third house two cases occurred within five days of each other; here the treatment was not well carried out at first, but there were three other children in the house who, after treatment was thoroughly attended to, did not take the disease. In a fourth house the treatment was not carried out at all at first, until three children had become infected. In another house the interval between the first and second case was nearly seven weeks. In the last house there was considerable doubt as to the second case being scarlet fever.

These results are not very conclusive as to the advantages of the treatment in view of the natural tendency of the disease to fluctuate from year to year; and it is clear that a longer trial is necessary for a judgment as to the applicability of the treatment among the general population not within institutions.

BIBLIOGRAPHY

Chapin. Quoted in Public Health, Nov., 1895.

Hospital Return. 1895.

Local Government Board. Memoranda for local arrangements relating to infectious disease. 1876. I. Hospital accommodation.

Cook, J. W. Annual Report for Tendring Rural District. 1909.

Johnstone, R. W. Report to Local Government Board on the Eton Rural District. 1899.

Low, J. Spencer. Report to Local Government Board on Hartley Wintney Rural District. 1907.

Millard, C. Killick. The value of Isolation Hospitals. Public Health, Nov., 1906.

Curgenven, J. B. On the use of oil of Eucalyptus Globulus in Scarlet Fever and other infectious diseases. Transactions of Epidemiological Society. 1889—90 and 1894—5.

Milne, R.   British Medical Journal, Oct. 31, 1908.
—— Transactions of Epidemiological Section, Royal Society of Medicine.
    1909—10.
—— A plea for the Home treatment and prevention of Scarlet Fever.
Park.   Annual Report for Borough of Dukinfield.   1910.   Quoted in Annual
    Report of County M.O.H. for Cheshire.   1910.
Gold, D. D.   The control and isolation of infectious diseases in thinly
    populated counties.   Public Health, May, 1912.

CHAPTER IV

AREAS TO BE SERVED BY AN ISOLATION HOSPITAL.
COMBINED AREAS

THE area which an isolation hospital may usefully serve will
depend partly upon the nature of the cases to be treated in it,
the patients in some diseases bearing removal better than those
in others, but also in part upon considerations of local topo-
graphy and means of transport.   If the area be too large the
usefulness of the hospital will be lessened owing to the difficulty
attending the conveyance of patients, especially those who are
seriously ill, over long distances, but on the other hand the
multiplication of small hospitals is to be avoided on grounds of
both economy and efficiency.   With the improvement in recent
years of means of communication, with the increasing readiness
to make use of hospitals in infectious illness, and with the
demand for better and therefore more costly accommodation
than the primitive structures and arrangements of former days,
the tendency has been towards enlarged areas and for combined
instead of small separate hospitals.

In the Sanitary Act, 1866, under which local authorities were
first given power to provide hospitals, this power was coupled
with the limitation "within the district"; and the power of
compulsory removal to hospital was similarly limited to a
hospital within the district, although two or more authorities
were empowered to combine in providing a common hospital.
As the earliest hospitals provided by local authorities were

temporary ones for cholera cases which cannot be moved far, the inconvenience of the limitation to the district may not have been obvious at first, but in view of the varying sizes and irregular shapes of many districts, and of the difficulty of obtaining suitable sites in the densely populated ones, it must have been perceived before very long, and the limitation was omitted in § 131, Public Health Act, 1875.

It was, however, formerly considered that in view of the terms of § 285, Public Health Act, 1875[1], a local authority was not empowered to erect a hospital in an adjoining district without the consent of the authority of that district, but this view was not sustained by the Court of Appeal in the case of Withington v. Manchester Corporation (62 Law J. Rep. Ch. D. 393, 1893). It is nevertheless undesirable for several reasons that a local authority should plant its hospital in the district of another authority if there is a suitable site available in its own ; and in cases where a local authority has sought sanction to a loan for the erection of a hospital outside its own district in that of an unwilling authority the late Local Government Board have required as a condition that the first authority shall be prepared to enter into an agreement, if so desired, for the reception into its hospital on reasonable terms of cases from the invaded district.

In crowded towns it may be difficult to find a sufficiently large and isolated site, at a reasonable cost, within the limits of the district, and this is especially so as regards small-pox hospital sites, which require to be placed far from populous localities. For this and other reasons a small-pox hospital may conveniently serve a larger area than that served by a hospital for the ordinary infectious diseases.

But even for other infectious diseases it is found that under present conditions a hospital may advantageously serve a larger area than was formerly supposed. From his experience

---

[1] § 285. Any local authority may, with the consent of the local authority of any adjoining district, execute and do in such adjoining district all or any of such works and things as they may execute and do within their own district, and on such terms as to payment and otherwise as may be agreed upon between them and the authority of the adjoining district.

Sir R. Thorne formed the opinion that a hospital should, if possible, be within the limits of the district for which it was intended, and that in order to be reasonably available it should, in the case of a town, be distant not much more than two miles, and in the case of a rural district not more than four or five miles from the populous parts of the district. He did not indeed find that removal for a distance of some five, or even seven or eight miles in a well-constructed ambulance, and over ordinarily good roads, had appeared to do harm to patients, provided their removal had been effected at an early stage of their illness, but he found that parents and friends assented much more readily to their removal to a hospital within easy distance than to a more distant one.

Dr J. Makinson Fox, writing also in 1882, expresses similar views in an address to the North Western Association of Medical Officers of Health. He says: "To seek to remove children further than an easy walking distance from their parents, during the time that they are suffering from acute and dangerous illnesses, is a course, however likely to secure the protection of the community, alike opposite to the requirements of the Statute, to the published teaching of its official expounders, and to the common instincts of humanity."

It is found, however, that with modern improvements in means of communication and transport, such as telephones, motor vehicles, and ambulances with india-rubber or pneumatic tyres and with the generally improved state of the roads, it is practicable to remove patients for longer distances than was the case 30 years ago, while with increased public appreciation of the advantages of hospital treatment the objection to removal of patients to a distance from their homes has in most parts of the country much diminished[1]. To a patient dangerously ill the mere act of removal involves an amount of added risk not lightly to be incurred; but it is the shifting of the patient

---

[1] There formerly existed in some parts of the country, especially in the manufacturing and mining districts, a strong aversion to entering hospitals of any kind—not only those for infectious disease—based apparently on ungrounded fears of ill-usage. This feeling, which is mentioned by Sir R. Thorne in connection with the non-use of the hospital at Aberdare, appears to have persisted in some districts in South Wales until quite recent years, and may not yet be wholly extinct.

rather than the actual distance traversed which constitutes the danger, and in a smoothly-running ambulance, over good roads, a mile or two more or less in the length of journey does not make any great difference to it.   In practice distances of 10 or 12 miles have not prevented the use of a hospital for cases of scarlet fever; while small-pox patients have on occasion been removed without harm by road for distances of 20 or even 30 miles[1].

Such distances, however, are to be regarded as indicating what is permissible with a view to avoid unnecessary multiplication of hospitals rather than as showing that distance and convenience of access are immaterial (see Chapter II).   Except London, there are few towns in England too large to be served by a single hospital for infectious diseases other than small-pox. The cities of Birmingham, Liverpool, Manchester, Sheffield and Leeds have each more than one such hospital; but in every instance either the additional hospital was originally erected for what was at the time a separate district but which has since been taken into the city, or else the erection of another hospital became necessary because more accommodation was required and there was not room to provide it on the original site.   Under the last mentioned circumstances, West Ham, in order to relieve the pressure on the Plaistow Hospital, has provided a convalescent home 10 miles distant in the country, to which scarlet fever patients when convalescent are transferred.

Similarly there are few rural districts in the country of an area too extensive to be served by a single centrally placed and conveniently accessible hospital.   In the case of the Isle of Wight

---

[1] " The larger the district (within certain limits) the greater the economy and the better the administration.   With too small a district the hospital is apt at times to be empty, which causes dissatisfaction on the score of apparently unnecessary expense. This was the case at Tolworth, but when the area was enlarged the objections ceased. It is true that the wider the area the greater will be the distance for some of the sick persons to be removed, but with good roads, such as those of Surrey, and with good ambulance arrangements, such as an efficient Hospital Board would easily provide, the consideration is practically insignificant.   The county medical officer of health has had experience which enables him to say emphatically that there is practically nothing whatever in this objection, which has been often raised and as often disposed of." From a Report on Isolation Hospital Accommodation in Surrey, by a Sub-Committee of the County Council, 1900.

Rural District, and of the Sevenoaks Rural District, certain groups of parishes, separated from the rest by distance or by a range of hills, were formed into hospital districts by orders of the respective County Councils under the Isolation Hospitals Act; and separate hospital accommodation has been provided for each portion of the district, either singly or jointly with other districts; but subsequent experience has seemed to show that a single hospital might have served the whole of each area with the included urban districts, and that there would have been a considerable saving of cost if that course had been adopted.

A large and populous borough may be expected to prefer to have a hospital of its own; and smaller districts in the neighbourhood may conveniently make arrangements for the reception into it of their cases of infectious disease, on terms which should be embodied in a formal agreement; but when neighbouring districts are of small area or population or of low rateable value, combination for the purpose of the joint provision and management of an isolation hospital is generally preferable; and it possesses distinct advantages, both as regards economy and efficiency, over the establishment of a separate hospital for each district. This is especially the case with small-pox hospitals; and in many instances, for the purpose of providing small-pox hospitals, separate combined areas have been formed, more extensive and embracing a larger number of districts than the areas formed for providing hospitals for other infectious diseases.

In the more rural parts of the country a market town with the surrounding rural area, or the whole of the districts comprised within one poor law Union, often form an area of a size and shape to be conveniently served, for infectious diseases other than small-pox, by a single hospital placed near the principal town. Very small isolation hospitals are not economical; unless a district is large enough to require accommodation for 12 to 14 patients, it should be required to join with one or more adjoining districts for the purpose of providing a joint isolation hospital.

The advantages of combination are thus set out in the late Local Government Board's Memorandum[1] "On the provision of Isolation Hospital accommodation by local authorities": "The

[1] Dated 1902.

unnecessary multiplication of small hospitals is to be avoided on grounds both of economy and of efficiency. As compared with that of several small hospitals the establishment of a single hospital containing an equal number of beds saves the cost of duplicating various buildings, appliances and officers, it facilitates the classification of patients according to the diseases from which they are suffering ; and it enables a more efficient staff to be maintained, since the hospital is less likely to remain empty for long periods." To these it may be added that a large part of the difficulty and expense involved in the establishment of a hospital for infectious diseases lies in the acquisition of a suitable site and its preparation for building; that in the case of a joint hospital there is only a single site to be acquired instead of several and the area for selection is larger; that the aggregate amount of land required is less, as a single larger site affords more facility for placing the hospital buildings in a proper relation to each other, the amount of space required for securing a proper distance of one building from another or from the boundary forming a less proportion of the whole area ; and that the length of fencing required to enclose a larger site is less in proportion to its area than that required to enclose a smaller area of similar shape. Thus if an area of one acre be required for a hospital of 8 beds, an area of 2 acres will suffice for one of more than 16 beds.

The objections raised by local authorities to combination for hospital provision are often based chiefly on local jealousies and the desire to retain their independence. It is sometimes alleged that there will be greater danger or injury to the district in which the hospital is placed if it receives cases from other districts than from the one district only; or that the conveyance of patients to it from outside districts will constitute a source of danger. Experience does not support these forebodings; except in the case of small-pox hospitals, the sites of which should be chosen so as to avoid this danger as far as possible, there is no evidence that infectious disease ever spreads from a well administered hospital at a proper distance from the boundary, and dwellings in the neighbourhood of such a hospital, even when separated from it only by the breadth of a street, have not shown any greater prevalence of disease than other parts of the district.

Nor is there any evidence that with ordinary care the conveyance of patients through the streets in a proper ambulance is any
danger to passers by, in the momentary exposure involved[1].

Another objection often raised is that the distance of the
hospital from outlying places in the combined district would
render it of no use to them, but they would nevertheless have to
contribute to its cost. The question of distance has already
been sufficiently referred to.

Again it is sometimes asserted that it will cost the district
more to take part in the establishment of a joint hospital
than to provide hospital accommodation separately for itself.
But for the reasons already given, assuming that the hospital
accommodation is of equal efficiency in the two cases, it should
cost the individual district less to provide it in combination than
separately, provided that due care and regard to economy in
the selection of the site and design and erection of the hospital
are exercised by the body charged with the work.

A frequent source of difficulty in effecting a combination of
districts for hospital purposes is the settling the proportion in
which the different districts shall contribute to the common fund
out of which the structural and establishment expenses of the
hospital are paid. The usual basis of apportionment is the
assessable value[2] of the respective districts, but in some instances
the basis adopted has been the respective populations of the
several districts at the last census, on the ground that the
use likely to be made of the hospital will be in proportion to
the number of inhabitants rather than to the assessable value.
Generally in a combination between an urban and a rural authority
in an agricultural county an apportionment on a basis of population would result in less being payable by the rural district
than would be the case if the apportionment were on a basis of
assessable value ; and hence the former is likely to be preferred
by rural district councils. On the other hand an objection to an

---

[1] See Chapter XI.

[2] The assessable value for the " general district rate " in an urban district, and for
" special expenses " in a rural district, differs from the rateable value for the relief of
the poor in that for the former tithes, land used as arable meadow or pasture ground
only or as woodlands, market gardens or nursery ground, land covered with water,
canals and railways, are assessed on only one-fourth of their net annual value. See
§§ 211, 1 (*b*) and 230, Public Health Act, 1875.

apportionment on the basis of population is that as the census is taken only once in ten years it may lead to an inequitable division of expenses towards the end of the period, where the population of one district is increasing rapidly and that of another is not. Occasionally by way of compromise the common fund has been apportioned one half on the basis of population and one half on that of assessable value.

There are several methods by which districts may combine for the purpose of providing a common hospital[1].

(*a*) Section 131, Public Health Act, 1875, gives in general terms the power to combine but does not set forth any particular method. The usual course is to appoint a joint committee for hospital purposes consisting of members of each authority, appointed under their general powers or under those of § 57, Local Government Act, 1894. The advantage of this informal mode of combination is that it can be carried out by the combining councils at once without waiting for Parliamentary sanction or for a County Council Order—a point which may be of advantage if temporary hospital accommodation is required on an emergency. The disadvantages are that such a joint committee has no legal status, and cannot hold land, enter into contracts, raise loans or expend money except as authorised by the councils appointing it, and if these councils are not agreed a deadlock may occur. Hence in some instances it has been found ultimately preferable to form a Joint Hospital Board.

(*b*) A Joint Hospital Board is formed under §§ 279—284, Public Health Act, 1875, by a provisional order issued now by the Ministry of Health after a local inquiry held by their inspectors, and subsequently confirmed by Parliament. The constitution and powers of the Joint Board and the proportion in which its expenses are to be defrayed are settled by the Ministry of Health in the provisional order. Upon the formation of a joint board the duties assigned to it cease to be exercisable by the individual authorities in the combined district, except by

---

[1] The several methods are more fully set forth in a memorandum on "Isolation Hospitals" issued by the late Local Government Board under date June 1910, which also sets out the steps necessary in order to obtain the Board's sanction to a loan for hospital purposes.

delegation from the joint board or where the joint board has omitted to carry them out. A joint board is a body corporate with power to hold lands, and can levy contributions, enter into contracts, and raise loans independently of the constituent authorities.

(*c*) Hospital districts under the Isolation Hospitals Acts are formed by Order of the County Council, who may be set in motion by a petition from one or more local authorities or from 25 or more ratepayers in any contributory place, or by a report from the county medical officer of health. A local inquiry is to be held by the County Council, and any local authority within the proposed hospital district objecting to its formation may appeal within three months to the Local Government Board[1]. When a hospital district has been formed by the County Council, a hospital committee is to be formed, consisting of representatives of the local areas in the district, with the addition, where the County Council make a contribution to the funds of the hospital, of members or representatives of that body. For further details the reader is referred to the Isolation Hospitals Acts, 1893 and 1901.

As between the formation of a Joint Hospital Board under the Public Health Act, and procedure under the Isolation Hospitals Act, 1893, as now amended by the Act of 1901, there is not in general much balance of advantage one way or the other. Where all parties are agreed an Order of the County Council can be obtained in less time than is necessary for the making and confirmation by Parliament of a provisional order; but on the other hand sanction to any loan required by a Hospital Committee under the Isolation Hospitals Act has to be obtained through the County Council, which may involve delay, and is subject to the limit of the County Council's borrowing powers; whereas a Joint Hospital Board has independent powers of borrowing irrespective of the amounts of debt of the constituent districts. A hospital district formed under the Isolation Hospitals Acts must be entirely within one administrative county, and no borough can be included without the consent of the Town Council, unless the population is under 10,000 and the Local Government Board[1] by order direct that the Act shall apply.

[1] Now the Ministry of Health.

The use of hospitals provided under the Isolation Hospitals Acts is limited to the notifiable infectious diseases, but may be extended to other diseases by Order. The formation of a hospital district under the Isolation Hospitals Acts does not abrogate the concurrent powers of the sanitary authority under the Public Health Acts.

The Isolation Hospitals Acts do not give the County Council direct power to establish or require the provision of a hospital ; they can only effect this, in the face of an unwilling authority, by constituting a hospital committee on which their own representatives preponderate, and in order to do this they must contribute in proportion to the cost of the hospital. But the powers which the County Council possess of contributing to the capital cost and current expenditure of hospitals which are constructed and managed to their satisfaction, enable them to exercise considerable influence towards the provision of hospitals and their maintenance in a due state of efficiency. These powers are extended by the Isolation Hospitals Act, 1901, so as to enable the County Council to contribute to hospitals established under the Public Health Act. The consent of the Ministry of Health is required to an annual contribution by a County Council to a hospital provided or extended otherwise than by means of loan. Hospitals provided under the Public Health Act may be transferred, under § 1, Isolation Hospitals Act, 1901, to the County Council of the district in which they are situated, for use under the Isolation Hospitals Acts.

BIBLIOGRAPHY

Memorandum of Medical Officer of Local Government Board "On the provision of Isolation Hospital Accommodation by Local Authorities." 1902.

Memorandum by Local Government Board on "Isolation Hospitals." June, 1910.

Isolation Hospitals Acts, 1893 and 1901.

Thorne. Hospital Report, and preface to reprint. 1901.

Parsons. Hospital Report. 1912.

Copnall, H. H. The Law relating to infectious diseases and Hospitals.

Fox, J. Makinson. The warrant and scope of infectious hospitals for the reception of non-paupers. Inaugural address to North Western Branch of Society of Medical Officers of Health. Warrington, 1882.
Barwise, S. Report on the Isolation Hospitals of Derbyshire. 1906.
—— Isolation Hospitals for small Urban and Rural Districts. Public Health, Feb., 1895.
Fosbroke, G. H. Removal of patients to Isolation Hospitals. Public Health, Feb., 1895.
Gold, D. D. The control and isolation of infectious diseases in thinly populated counties. Public Health, May, 1912.

CHAPTER V

SITES FOR ISOLATION HOSPITALS

THE selection of a suitable site for an isolation hospital is a matter of great importance, not only as regards the usefulness and convenience of working of the hospital, but also from the point of view of economy, as an ill-chosen site may add greatly to the cost of erection of the hospital. It is not merely that the site may be unnecessarily large, or the price per acre unduly high ; but that the site may be difficult of access, or the ground of an unsuitable character, or costly preliminary works of drainage, water supply, or road-making may be needed in order to adapt it for building on. All these things add largely to the cost of a hospital over and above the price of the land. Indeed, it may be true economy to pay a larger total sum or a higher price per acre for a good site than to buy cheaply one which will require a large further expenditure upon it, or involve increased expense in maintenance. Unfortunately, the matter is not one which local authorities have much in their own hands, for owing to the alarm and dislike which the idea of an infectious hospital inspires, owners of what is regarded as " eligible building land," or of land in the vicinity of a town where facilities exist for connecting with public services, are commonly unwilling to sell it for hospital purposes, for fear of depreciating the rest of their property. Hence, in order to get a site at all, local authorities may be obliged to buy a larger and more costly one than they require, or one remote from public water supply or sewers ; or in other respects not so good as they might wish.

It is indeed possible for a local authority to acquire power under the Lands Clauses Acts for the compulsory purchase of land for hospital purposes, but the necessary procedure involves so much uncertainty, delay and expense, that this course is only to be resorted to as a last resource.

The following are the recommendations of the late Local Government Board with respect to the choice of a hospital site:— " In selecting a site for an isolation hospital the following considerations should be had in view :—It should be convenient of access, and, as far as practicable, central for the population and area which it is to serve ; but of course not in a very populous neighbourhood. (In the case of hospitals in which small-pox is intended to be received the choice of site must be specially governed by considerations as to the number of inhabitants in the neighbourhood, which will be referred to later on.) It will be of much convenience if sewers and a public water service are available; but, if not, a sufficient supply of wholesome water must be provided, and arrangements will have to be made for the treatment of the sewage by application to land, due care being taken to avoid pollution of any well or spring or of any river. The site should be in a healthy and open situation with a dry subsoil, and should be preferably of a compact and regular shape, and not too steep. Its area will depend upon the size of the hospital, and, except in the case of a very small hospital, should rarely be less than two acres ; indeed it is well to obtain a larger site than may at first be required, in order to afford space for subsequent extension if necessary. More land, too, will be needed if the sewage has to be disposed of on the site."

The approval of a site by the Ministry of Health is, however, only required when sanction to a loan is sought, or when, for some other reason, the Ministry's approval of a hospital is needed. In other cases the selection rests with the hospital authority themselves, subject to the liability not to cause a nuisance.

In cases in which the sanction of the Ministry of Health is needed, the Ministry require as a condition that every building intended to contain infected persons or articles shall be distant at least 40 feet from the boundary of the site, and there should be a similar distance between each such building and any other.

The Ministry further require that the site, or so much of it as is to form the hospital curtilage, shall be enclosed in such a way that there shall be a screen and barrier sufficient to prevent illicit communication between patients in the hospital and persons outside. Ordinarily a wall, or close fence, at least 6 feet 6 inches high, is required, this height being necessary in order to prevent people looking over it; but in isolated situations, on sides to which there is no public right of way, the fence may consist of a hedge or belt of shrubs between two rows of open unclimbable railings, or barbed wire. The object of these requirements is to prevent any risk of spread of infection from the hospital to persons outside, and the fact that they are insisted on should tend to obviate local objections to the establishment of an isolation hospital as a danger to the neighbourhood. The fencing of hospital sites is always a serious item of expense. For satisfying the requirements of the Ministry of Health as to a close fence 6 feet 6 inches high, the cheapest and most serviceable type is probably the recognised form of close galvanised iron or wood fencing. The enclosure of a 4 acre plot with galvanised iron fencing was estimated, in 1919, at 11s. 9d. per yard making a total of £358; while a cleft oak fence at 16s. 6d. per yard cost £503. To enclose the same site with a 6 feet 6 inches brick wall at 39s. per yard was estimated in 1919 to cost £1190. But it is possible that these prices will be reduced when times become more normal.

Sir R. Thorne's inquiries tended to show that in well administered hospitals, having an open space of some 40 feet between the hospital wards and any neighbouring thoroughfares or dwellings, no risk of the spread of infection from scarlet fever, typhus, and enteric fever need be apprehended, and this conclusion was confirmed by the results of an investigation made at the London Fever Hospital, Islington, by Mr (now Sir Shirley) Murphy, and extending over a long series of years, during which large numbers of typhus, relapsing, enteric and scarlet fever patients had been treated at a hospital surrounded on all sides with a not inconsiderable population residing in houses at a distance varying from 49 to 80 feet from the wards. Among this population not a single case of typhus or relapsing fever could be heard of, and though there had been certain cases of scarlet and enteric fever the number was not greater than might be expected according to the prevalence of these diseases in London generally. The Royal Commission on Small-pox and Fever Hospitals in 1882 said :

"All evidence goes to show that well-conducted fever hospitals (as opposed to those for small-pox) involve no appreciable risk to the neighbourhood."

It is not contended that a distance less than 40 feet would necessarily entail danger of spread of infection, but it having been found advisable to make a rule on the subject, a distance of 40 feet was adopted on the above grounds, as having been in practice found sufficient to secure safety.

The need for a sufficient fence has been shown by experience. More than one outbreak of small-pox has been caused by the escape of delirious patients from hospital. An open fence to which there is access on both sides, may allow of contact between convalescent patients and their friends on the other side, and the passing of infected articles outwards, and of spirits and other contraband articles inwards. Nurses at insufficiently fenced hospitals have sometimes been molested by tramps.

Area of site. The area required will depend upon the size of the hospital to be erected. The late Local Government Board recommended that the number of patients should not exceed 20 per acre, but the requirement of a 40-foot zone between the wards and the boundary generally entails a less number of beds. It is obvious that the 40-foot zone will occupy a greater proportion of the area of a very small site than of a larger one, and for this reason, and to allow of future extensions which may be needed, it is desirable to obtain more than a bare sufficiency of space. Any portion of it not intended at first to be used for hospital purposes need not be included in the boundary fence.

It is advisable that the nature of the ground on which buildings are to be erected, and in the sewage disposal area, should be ascertained by trial holes. Much expense has sometimes been caused by foundations having to be constructed on wet and treacherous ground, or on the filled-up and forgotten sites of old excavations.

The most favourable aspect for wards being S.E., a site

which slopes in that direction is preferable. Regard must also be had to the need for a fall for drainage, and where the sewage has to be disposed of on the site, an additional area of land conveniently situated will be required for the purpose. The sewage disposal area should be not smaller than at the rate of an acre for every hundred persons whom the hospital will be capable of containing. The mode of disposal may be by any approved modern method which may be most suitable under the circumstances, but care must be taken that the effluent shall not pollute any stream, or any well or other water source used for drinking purposes.

Earth closets have not been found suitable for hospital use, owing to the amount of liquid to be disposed of, and the difficulty of securing a regular supply of suitable dry earth, and daily removal of their contents. Cesspools are to be avoided owing to the expense and offensiveness of their periodical emptying and the nuisance apt to arise in the disposal of their contents. The volume of waste liquid produced at a hospital is large owing to the amount of washing required ; it is estimated at 40 to 50 gallons per head per day. Hence a site which allows of drainage into public sewers is to be preferred to one where sewage would have to be treated on the site itself, even if the former should cost somewhat more.

Objections are sometimes raised to the discharge of the sewage from an infectious hospital into the public sewers on the ground that it may spread disease. Experience however does not support this objection ; in many places hospital sewage is discharged into the sewers, and there appears to be no evidence of ill-effects having arisen from the practice. Experiments have shown that sewage is not a favourable medium for the multiplication of specific pathogenic organisms, such as those of enteric fever and cholera, and their life in it is very limited. The less specific organisms, such as streptococci and bacillus enteritidis sporogenes, survive in sewage and even in the effluent after bacterial treatment; but these are found in all sewage, whether from a hospital or not. The highly resistant spores of the bacillus of anthrax will also live in sewage and survive treatment, but these are not likely to be met with in the sewage from an isolation hospital. The liability to contain pathogenic organisms attaches to all domestic sewage, and the danger from it should be guarded against ; but there is no reason to suppose that it is increased by the admission of sewage from an isolation hospital. In a few instances sterilising tanks have been constructed for sterilising the hospital sewage in bulk by steam or chemical disinfectants, but their use appears unnecessary, and has usually in course of time been abandoned.

Sites near Sewage Farms, etc. Owing to the difficulty of obtaining land for hospital purposes, local authorities are sometimes obliged to be content with sites in proximity to establishments and places the neighbourhood of which is considered undesirable for residences, as sewage works[1], cemeteries[2], or destructors[3]. Two isolation hospitals on the outskirts of London adjoin main lines of railway along which heavy trains are constantly passing at a high rate of speed. While a site free from such drawbacks is to be preferred, it does not appear that in practice they interfere materially with the usefulness and efficiency of the hospital; and where local authorities and their medical advisers have been satisfied that the surroundings of a site did not preclude its use the late Local Government Board generally did not refuse to sanction it on such grounds, though in two instances they refused to sanction loans for the purchase of hospital sites which they were advised by H. M. Inspector of Explosives were within the zone of danger from a powder magazine[4].

At the Warwick Joint Hospital, which is 150 yards from the nearest irrigated part of the Leamington sewage farm, Dr George Wilson, former medical officer of health, has stated that a bad smell is occasionally perceived when the pumping of sewage is first started in the morning, but that the proximity of the sewage farm has neither injured the patients or staff, nor detracted from the usefulness or

---

[1] *E.g.* Ealing, Brentford, Wimbledon, Croydon borough, Watford, Warwick, West Bromwich (small-pox hospital).

[2] *E.g.* Wimbledon, Norwich, Middlesbrough.

[3] *E.g.* Acton.

[4] The Local Government Board consider it undesirable that an isolation hospital site should be so near a workhouse as to suggest an association with poor relief.

popularity of the hospital[1]. At one isolation hospital, however, serious nuisance has been occasioned by the formation of a tip for town refuse close by, and at another from the proximity of an abattoir and piggeries; both of these places would be especially objectionable as breeding places for flies, which might convey infection.

As regards the power to use for the purpose of a hospital for infectious diseases surplus land acquired for the purpose of a sewage farm, reference should be made to the case of the Attorney-General *v.* Hanwell Urban District Council, Court of Appeal, June 20th, 1900; in which it was held that surplus land which had been compulsorily acquired for the purpose of sewage disposal could not be used by the District Council for the purposes of a permanent isolation hospital, and that the Local Government Board had no power to give a direction under § 175, Public Health Act, 1875, that it should be so used. This power was, however, given to the Board by § 95, Public Health Acts Amendment Act, 1907, if put in force in the district, but before giving such a direction in the case of a hospital for infectious diseases the Board[2] must cause a public inquiry to be held into the matter. The use as a site for a temporary hospital of the unappropriated portion of land purchased for a cemetery, requires, under § 6, Burial Act, 1900, the consent of the Ministry of Health, if the site has been formally approved by the Ministry for use as a cemetery.

Apart from such a case, or from a breach of covenant[3], there appears to be no legal power to prevent the use for the purposes of an isolation hospital of a particular site, unless a nuisance has actually arisen.

In the case of the Fulham and Hampstead hospitals of the Metropolitan Asylums Board, injunctions were issued by the Courts restraining the use of those hospitals for small-pox, that disease having been found to spread around them—see

[1] At Berlin several large sanatoria for tuberculosis patients and convalescents have been established on the area of the sewage farms. It is however desirable that such places should be in the purest air obtainable.

[2] Now Ministry of Health.

[3] The Courts have held that covenants in leases, whereby the lessee undertook not to carry on upon the premises any trade or business, or not to do anything which should be a nuisance or annoyance to the neighbourhood, prohibited the use of the premises as a hospital or sanatorium.

Chapter IX—and in the case of Chapman and wife *v.* Gillingham Urban District Council (reported in *Public Health*, May, 1903) damages were obtained by the plaintiffs for the death of their daughter and the illness of other persons from small-pox, by reason of the use of a stable 200 yards from the plaintiffs' house as a temporary small-pox hospital, and for conducting it in a negligent manner. On the other hand, in the cases of Attorney-General *v.* Guildford, Godalming, and Woking Joint Hospital Board (1896), of Harrop *v.* Mayor, etc., of Ossett (1898), and of Attorney-General *v.* Mayor, etc., of Nottingham (1904), injunctions against the use of particular sites for the purpose of small-pox hospitals were refused where no actual case of injury had arisen and the action was merely *quia timet.* In the last case Mr Justice Farwell said : " To sustain the injunction the law requires proof by the plaintiff of a well-founded apprehension of injury—proof of actual and real danger—a strong probability almost amounting to moral certainty, that if the hospital be established it will be an actionable nuisance. A sentiment of danger and dislike however natural and justified ; certainty that the hospital will be disagreeable or inconvenient ; proof that it will abridge a man's pleasure or make him anxious ; the inability of the Court to say that no danger will arise ; none of these, accompanied by depreciation of property, will discharge the burden of proof which rests on the plaintiffs, or justify a merely precautionary injunction, restraining an owner's use of his own land upon the ground of apprehended nuisance to his neighbours." " An isolation hospital reduces the risk for every inhabitant of the district. It is in fact a necessity, and though the individual must be protected the public advantage must not be forbidden, unless the danger and injury to the individual are clearly proved."

In the High Court of Dublin, however, an injunction has been given beforehand against the use of a hospital for small-pox and other infectious diseases near a village, on the ground of anticipated danger (*Public Health*, August, 1903).

Drs Gregory and Marson of the London Small-pox Hospital, advised that a small-pox ward should not be within 150 feet of any dwelling-house or public road—see evidence of Dr Munk before the Royal Commission on Small-Pox and Fever Hospitals; see also chapter on small-pox hospitals.

> In view of the frequently demonstrated liability of small-pox hospitals to disseminate that disease to neighbouring communities, and in order to lessen the risk of such occurrence, the Local Government Board, now the Ministry of Health, require the following conditions to be complied with in the case of small-pox hospitals provided by means of loans sanctioned by them :—
>
> 1st. The site must not have within a quarter of a mile of it either a hospital, whether for infectious diseases or not, or a workhouse, asylum, or any similar establishment, or a population of as many as 200 persons.
>
> 2nd. The site must not have within half a mile of it a population of as many as 600 persons, whether in one or more institutions, or in dwelling-houses.
>
> 3rd. Even where the above conditions are fulfilled, a hospital must not be used at one and the same time for the reception of cases of small-pox and of any other class of disease.

BIBLIOGRAPHY

Memorandum of Local Government Board on Isolation Hospitals.
Report of Hospitals Commission. 1882.
Thorne. Hospital Report. 1882.
Parsons. Hospital Report. 1912.
Lawes and Andrewes. Report to London County Council on Micro-organisms of Sewage. December, 1894.
Glaister. Text-book of Public Health. Edinburgh. 1910.
Copnall. The Law relating to Infectious Diseases and Hospitals. 1899.

CHAPTER VI

DESIGN OF ISOLATION HOSPITALS

THE most essential portion of a hospital is of course the wards for the reception of patients, but since it is necessary to the welfare of the sick that they should be provided with food and attendance and in other respects properly cared for, there must be, in addition to the ward-blocks, administrative accommodation containing kitchen, storage for food, linen and other requisites, and quarters for staff, and also laundry and other out-offices. There are thus required in every hospital, however small, three departments, viz. ward-block or blocks, administration, and out-offices, and these should be in separate buildings[1]. There should also usually be separate ward blocks for different infectious diseases. But the accessory buildings which are necessary even for a hospital containing very few beds will suffice, at any rate without proportional increase in size or cost, for a larger one, containing say double the number of beds, and so on up to a point at which duplication becomes necessary. By way of illustration a hospital containing only two beds, in two single-bed wards, might require if there were in it patients who were seriously ill, at least one day nurse and a night nurse, for whom accommodation would have to be provided, but the same number of nurses might suffice if the wards contained four beds each, *i.e.* eight in all. If a second 8-bed block were added the number of nurses who might require housing would be doubled, but one caretaker would still suffice, and so with other matters.

Hence in very small hospitals the cost, divided by the number of beds, works out to a high figure and the multiplication of such hospitals involves unnecessary expense, where by a combination of districts a single hospital can be made to serve. In arranging a hospital scheme a minimum number of 12—20 beds should, unless under exceptional circumstances, be aimed at, and a larger number is generally preferable. The size which is desirable for an isolation hospital finds a maximum limit when the hospital becomes too large for the administrative superintendence (apart from the treatment of the patients) to be effectually carried out by one medical superintendent. This size has sometimes been placed at 300 beds; but this number is exceeded in the hospitals of the Metropolitan Asylums Board and other modern hospitals.

[1] In two or three districts of very small population and rateable value, where combination with any other district appeared impracticable, small isolation hospitals have been erected by means of loans sanctioned by the late Local Government Board in which, for the sake of cheapness, the three departments are placed in a single block; the wards, nurses' quarters and washhouse being separately entered from the open air under a verandah. See plans of Lydd and Sedbergh Hospitals, Chapter XIX. A somewhat similar plan was formerly issued by the Local Government Board, but has not been adopted in many instances.

As regards the size of the hospital in relation to the population for which it is to serve, the usual estimate is one bed for every 1000 persons, but for reasons already mentioned (see p. 37) the requirements of different districts in this respect will vary with local circumstances. The proportion of one bed to 1000 persons (in addition to provision for small-pox) seems to have been first suggested by the late Sir G. Buchanan in the annual oration delivered before the Medical Society of London in 1875, but it has not been insisted on by the late Local Government Board, nor has it been their practice to refuse to sanction loans for hospitals which did not afford this proportion of beds, provided that the site were of sufficient area, and that the buildings which it was proposed to erect were so placed and planned as to admit of extension, if found to be needed at a later date.

Facility for future extension, permanent or temporary, is indeed a point of much importance and one which should always be borne in mind in designing a hospital, and especially in designing the administration block. Many of the earlier isolation hospitals were subsequently found by experience to be deficient in accommodation for the nursing staff required, and where the administration block was not planned so as to admit of easy extension, the providing of further accommodation has entailed much expense, either in large alterations to the existing building or in erecting another block. An additional number of beds for patients can usually be more easily provided, where there is room on the site, by lengthening existing wards or by building new blocks, but it must be borne in mind that any considerable addition to the number of beds will probably involve the need for more nurses, for whom quarters must be provided.

A site purchased for hospital purposes sometimes has on it buildings which it is desired to utilise. But, as pointed out in the late Local Government Board's Memorandum, existing buildings originally designed for a different purpose, such as dwelling houses, even when of large size, are rarely found to be well adapted for the reception of patients; especially for the accommodation at one time of patients suffering from different infectious diseases. An existing house, however, may sometimes serve as the administration-block, if it have sufficient land attached on which to erect ward-blocks. Stables and other outbuildings may also sometimes be adapted for use for a laundry or an ambulance shed.

With a view to maintaining due supervision and control over the persons entering and leaving the hospital there should be no unnecessary entrances to the curtilage. If a second entrance to the laundry block is needed for such purposes as carting in coals, or bringing articles from outside for disinfection, it should be closed by doors which can be kept locked when not in use.

The administration block should be so placed as to command the entrance to the hospital; but at hospitals of any considerable size it will be found convenient to have a porter's lodge near the gate, which may form the residence for a man employed about the hospital. In connection with this may be provided a waiting-room for visitors, and discharging rooms for convalescent patients[1].

The administration block should be kept free from patients and infected articles, and should contain quarters for the matron or caretaker, and a sufficient number of bedrooms for the nurses and servants who will be required to work the hospital when in full operation; also a nurses' sitting room, a kitchen (preferably in a one-storey projection with top ventilation), store rooms, dispensary, etc.[2] In hospitals of considerable size, say 50 beds and upwards, separate apartments for a resident medical officer containing a bedroom and sitting room will also be necessary. It is well to provide in the administration block accommodation on a scale somewhat in excess of what may be at first required, in order that it may be available for future extensions of the hospital, temporary or permanent; but in any case the block should be so planned that it can be easily enlarged in the future if necessary. This is generally most conveniently done by

---

[1] It is not advisable that the porter's lodge should contain accommodation for a family of children.

[2] "The Administration Block (including a competent matron, superintendent and staff) has been compared to the engine which drives the machinery on which the working of the hospital depends. It forms a good part of the cost, but it is absolutely essential." *Report on Isolation Hospital Accommodation in Surrey* by a Sub-Committee of the County Council, 1900.

placing the bedrooms along the sides of a corridor, which can be extended in length when it is necessary to provide more rooms. A special set of bedrooms may be usefully provided in a quiet part of the block with a shady aspect, where the night nurses may sleep undisturbed by day. At very large hospitals a separate block for the nurses' home is sometimes provided. It is desirable that the caretaker's quarters, if in the administration block, should be distinct from those of the nurses.

If the building is of more than two storeys in height special means of escape from the upper storey in case of fire should be provided. There should be a sufficient number of bath rooms conveniently accessible, usually one on each floor, and a lavatory on the ground floor where nurses may wash, on coming in from the wards ; and generally the block should be furnished, with a view to saving labour, with the conveniences usual in a large and well arranged dwelling house. There should be ample storage room for food, groceries, medical stores and household and bed-linen ; and the linen store may appropriately be placed near the hot water system of pipes. In large hospitals the administration block should be connected by telephone with the several ward blocks, and wherever possible the hospital should be connected through the general telephone system with the offices of the District Council and the residence of the medical attendant, so as to facilitate enquiries by parents, and calling the doctor in an emergency. Section 13, Isolation Hospitals Act, 1893, prescribes that every isolation hospital shall so far as practicable be in connection with the system of telegraphs, but telephonic communication might no doubt be held to meet this requirement.

The disposition of the other buildings on the site will be largely governed by its shape and contour. They should be sufficiently far apart to allow of free access of light and circulation of air, and to permit of any future extension likely to be necessary, and buildings intended to contain patients or infected articles should be at least 40 ft. from any other building and from the boundary fence. The distance between any two ward blocks should be at least twice the height of the blocks. On the other hand if the buildings are too scattered on the site, the work of the hospital staff is increased, as is also the cost of roadmaking and of the necessary connections with the drainage and water supply.

Many of the earlier isolation hospitals had corridors or covered ways connecting the administration block with the ward blocks, but these are not now generally considered necessary except on very bleak sites. Where provided they may consist of a covered way, open at the sides, and with a central screen not reaching to the roof.

Subways between the blocks for the conveyance of pipes and wires are useful, especially where there is a system of heating from a central boiler, as described in the next chapter.

The ward-blocks, for convenience of administration, are usually one-storey buildings, except at large hospitals or where

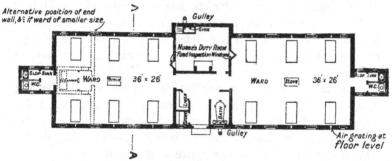

Fig. 1. Showing plan C of the late Local Government Board's model.

exigencies of space necessitate the erection of two-storey buildings. In such cases each storey should be separately entered from the outer air, and access to the upper floor should be by a fireproof staircase, and if possible by a lift capable of carrying patients.

In almost all modern hospitals, whether for infectious diseases or other purposes, the main wards are built on the pavilion plan with windows on opposite sides. At the Victoria Hospital, Belfast, a general hospital, the wards, for economy of space, are placed contiguously side by side, and are lighted from the roof and by a window at one end, and are ventilated artificially on the plenum principle. This system is said to be satisfactory in the particular instance, but does not appear to present any advantage in the case of an isolation hospital.

P.

6

An isolation hospital, other than the very smallest, will need ward-blocks of two kinds, some of the pavilion form, exemplified by plan C (see Fig. 1, p. 81) in the Local Government Board's Memorandum, for patients suffering from one disease, this being the plan on which a number of such patients may be most cheaply housed and most conveniently attended to; and others with small separate single-bed or two-bed wards, preferably separately entered from the open air, in which cases of different diseases may, with proper precautions in nursing, be treated at the same time without serious risk of interchange of infection. Such a block— often called an "isolation," "observation" or "cubicle" block— serves for the classification of patients in various ways, *e.g.* for the segregation of a patient who develops a second infectious disease (mixed infection), for the keeping under observation of a doubtful case, or for a case which proves not to be of an infectious nature. It may also be used, instead of the larger pavilion block, on the occasion of an outbreak of infectious disease comprising only a few cases, or for a few cases of a second disease, when the pavilion is already in use for one disease, or for keeping a convalescent patient apart for a few days before his discharge. Hence although in blocks of this kind, the cost of construction per bed is somewhat higher and administration somewhat less convenient than in a block on the pavilion plan, the beds can be used under a greater variety of circumstances, and the same number of beds will go farther in blocks on the separate principle than in pavilions.

In hospitals not on a very large scale the wards intended for the reception of a number of patients suffering from the same disease are generally in pairs, a ward for each sex, the centre of the block between the two wards being occupied by the nurses' duty room, bathroom, etc. as in the official plan C (Fig. 1, p. 81). Sometimes the wards are made of unequal sizes as indicated in the plan, on the ground that young children of both sexes may occupy the same ward with adult females.

The space above the centre of the block may be utilised for a day room for convalescents. As the height of the duty room need not be more than 9 ft. while that of the wards is 13 ft., the construction of a room in the spare space costs comparatively little: and it can be sufficiently lighted by windows in gable walls at the front and back. Such a room has been found very useful, especially in scarlet fever blocks, as a place where convalescent children can play without disturbing patients who are still in the acute stage, and where they will be out of the infected air of the ward. For this latter reason the convalescent room should preferably be approached by stairs from the open air under a porch. In large hospitals where several pavilions may be required for cases of a single disease, a pavilion may consist of a single large ward, with the duty room, etc. at one end, and this arrangement may be repeated on the first floor if the building is of two storeys. It is not generally advisable however that the number of beds in a ward should exceed 20.

The water-closets and slop-sinks are placed in annexes separated aerially from the wards by intervening cross-ventilated lobbies. These are commonly placed at the farther ends of the wards; but a position at the side of the wards, though it occupies more space on the ground, is sometimes preferred as more conveniently central, and also where a future extension of the wards in length is contemplated, as an annexe at the end of the ward would in that case have to be removed and rebuilt. Where owing to the large number of beds in the wards a separate bath for each ward is necessary one or both may be placed in a bathroom in a similar position ; but a cross-ventilated lobby is not necessary in the case of a bathroom.

Small wards suitable for the separate treatment of special or doubtful cases should be provided in the proportion of at least one for every ten beds in the hospital. There are various ways in which they may be arranged.

Thus single-bed wards may be annexed to the main wards in a pavilion block, as shown in the "alternative plan" with the official plan C (see p. 84, Figs. 2 and 3).

These are useful for special cases of the same disease as that treated in the main wards, e.g., for delirious patients, for septic cases or cases requiring operation, or for private patients for whom separate accommodation is desired, but are not intended for cases of a different disease. A greater degree of aerial separation can be got by making the entrance through an intervening lobby, instead of direct from the main wards, but in that case the wards project farther, and may interfere to some extent with the light to windows on that side of the block. (See plan of Colne and Holme Joint Hospital in Chapter XIX.) The single-bed wards may be entered from the nurse's duty room instead of from the main wards by substituting a glazed door

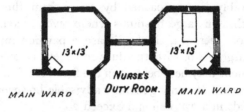

Fig. 2.   Showing alternative plan with plan C, for separation rooms.

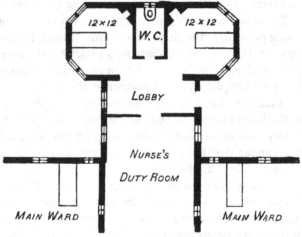

Fig. 3.   Showing separation wards as at Lincoln Isolation Hospital.

for the inspection windows shown in the official plan, or may be placed at the back of the duty room as in the alternative plan Fig. 3 above.

The space above the centre of a pavilion block has sometimes been utilised for small wards.

The small wards may form a separate block, as in the official plans B and D (see Figs. 4 and 6, pp. 85 and 86), in which each ward is entered separately from the open air under a verandah.

In plan B each ward contains two beds, as affording more accommodation on occasions when the ward may be used for one or two cases of a disease different from that under treatment in the main block, but in plan D they are of a size only for a single bed. In this plan the partitions between the wards are of plate glass, for the purpose of facilitating supervision from the duty room; it is found also that children, who are apt to feel lonely and

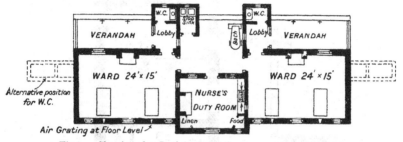

Fig. 4. Showing plan B of the Local Government Board's model.

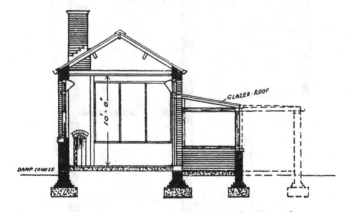

Fig. 5. Showing section through ward, plan D, p. 86.

frightened in a room by themselves, are contented if they can see other patients.

There may be a number of single-bed wards or compartments separated by glazed partitions within the main walls of one large block, either in a double row, each compartment being entered separately from the open air under a verandah, as at the Walthamstow, Croydon Borough, and Norwich Hospitals, or in

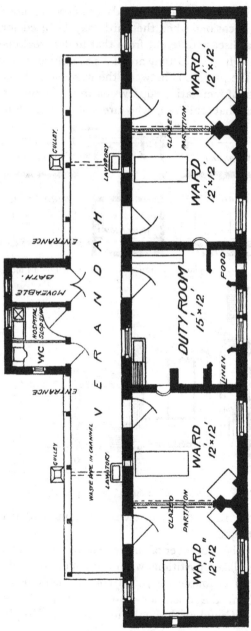

Fig. 6. Showing plan D of the Local Government Board's model.

a row on each side of a central corridor, as at the Eastern
Hospital of the Metropolitan Asylums Board, the East Ham
Hospital and the Pasteur Hospital at Paris. (See Chapter XIX.)
In the above instances there is complete aerial disconnection
between one compartment and another, or they are connected
only by a corridor, but at the South Western Hospital of the
Metropolitan Asylums Board, at Stockwell, a large ward has
been divided into a number of cubicles by glazed partitions
which do not reach to the ceiling of the ward. The arrangement
is described in detail by Dr Caiger, medical superintendent, in a
paper read before the Society of Medical Officers of Health on
April 7th, 1911, and published in *Public Health* for June, 1911,
from which the following extract is taken:

"Each of these two wards, which before conversion into cubicles contained
18 beds, is 100 feet in length and 28 feet broad. It is divided by glass partitions,
framed in iron, with a white enamelled surface, reaching to a height of 7 feet above
the floor level, into 16 cubicles.

"A central passage, 5 feet 6 inches wide, runs the whole length of the ward,
intersected at its middle point by a transverse passage of the same width leading
to the bath rooms and sanitary annexe, one on each side of the ward. A row of
cubicles is placed on either side of the central passage, the doorways of which,
however, are not placed immediately opposite each other, but are arranged on the
'hit and miss' principle.

"The cubicle doors are only 3 feet 6 inches in height, the upper portion
of the door opening being entirely unenclosed. These stable doors are double
hung and fitted with spring hinges to enable them to swing in either direction.
They readily open with the pressure of the toe or knee, thereby obviating the
necessity of the nurse handling them in passing through, and she thus has both
hands free for carrying things in and out of the cubicles.

"The proportion of floor space per bed is 175 square feet, and of this about
120 square feet are enclosed within the cubicle. The height of the ward being
14 feet, the total cubic space is 2450 feet per bed—or 2100 cubic feet, reckoned
on the 12-foot basis.

"The ward is ventilated as a whole by means of large-winged fanlights over
the windows, and the partitions are so disposed as to provide each cubicle with
a separate window. Under every window is a fresh-air inlet, opening behind a
double row of low-pressure hot-water pipes running round the ward. Additional
warming is provided by means of four open fireplaces in the centre of the ward.

"Each cubicle is furnished with a fixed lavatory basin, the waste pipe from
which is carried through the wall, and discharges over an open gully in the airing
court. Over it is fixed a tepid spray, worked by a pedal action.

"The only furniture allowed in the cubicle in addition to the bed or cot is a
bed locker and a bent-wood arm-chair. The locker is made of enamelled iron,
and has a plate-glass top and one shelf of the same material.

" Separate linen overalls are provided in each of the cubicles. These are hung on movable brass hooks, and are worn by the medical officer and nurse when attending to that particular patient, while a sterilised towel, hung in proximity to the spray, affords a convenient opportunity for the ablution and drying of the hands immediately before leaving the cubicle.

" The bath room attached to each of the wards is furnished with a portable enamelled iron bath, which can easily be run into the cubicles, if desired; and a gas-heated copper steriliser, provided with a hot-water supply and a fixed waste, provides facilities for sterilising every article which has been used for the patient's treatment.

" On the side of the ward opposite to the bath room is the lavatory annexe, containing a w.c., bed-pan flush, and a scalding sink for the efficient cleansing of utensils.

" In the scullery serving the ward is a second steriliser of larger size for the disinfection of plates, cups, mugs, tumblers, knives, forks and spoons, etc., when removed from the cubicles after use by any of the patients.

" Attached to each of the wards, and opening into the ward-lobby, is a 'separation' room, containing two beds. It is provided with a separate w.c., slop sink and lavatory basins for the use of the patients occupying it."

In this arrangement there is cross-ventilation of the whole ward, and each cubicle shares in it. Rooms in a single row, as in the Local Government Board plans B and D (Figs. 4 and 6), can also be cross-ventilated from windows on either side. But with compartments in a double row there is more difficulty and some special arrangement is necessary. At the Eastern Hospital of the Metropolitan Asylums Board a 20-bed ward, Temperance Ward, has been converted into an isolation ward, by dividing it by glazed partitions into 20 separate chambers. The ground plan is similar to that of the cubicle wards at the South Western Hospital, but the partitions are carried up to the ceiling, so that the chambers are completely separated from one another, except that they are entered from the central corridor. They have no cross-ventilation by windows, but an artificial system of ventilation is installed. They are described and figured by Dr Goodall in the annual report of the Metropolitan Asylums Board for 1910.

At Walthamstow Hospital there are large stoneware pipes, opening near the ground level on one side of the block, and passing under the floor of the nearer compartment to a perforated box on the floor of the compartment on the opposite side of the block; there is also an outlet opening in the ceiling of each compartment. At the Croydon Borough Hospital a slanting duct runs from the top of each compartment to an opening on the opposite slope of the roof, see Chapter XIX.

It will be seen that there are three different systems varying in the degree of aerial separation between the several compartments.

1st. Each compartment is completely separated from any other, and is separately entered from the open air under a verandah, as at the Walthamstow and Croydon Hospitals and in the Board's plan D.

2nd. Each compartment is separated from any other by a partition reaching to the ceiling, but the compartments are all entered from one corridor, as in the Pasteur Hospital and

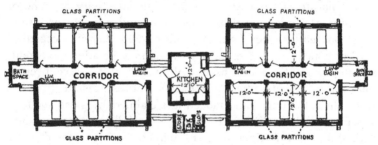

Fig. 6 a. East Ham Hospital. Isolation block with separate compartments for each patient.

Hospital for Sick Children at Paris, and at East Ham Isolation Hospital (see Fig. 6 a), and the Eastern Hospital of the Metropolitan Asylums Board.

3rd. The compartments or cubicles are all entered from one corridor and are separated from one another only by partitions not reaching to the ceiling, as at the South Western Hospital.

Whether one or another of these arrangements is to be preferred depends largely upon the mode in which infection is assumed to be spread in the diseases intended to be treated in the hospital. If the contagion is only conveyed attached to things such as nurses' hands, instruments and articles of furniture ("mediate infection") or by droplets expelled in coughing etc. reaching another patient point blank ("droplet infection") the partial separation afforded in a cubicle incompletely partitioned off may suffice, but if the infection is capable of being diffused more widely through the air complete separation will be necessary for safety.   Dr Caiger's experience goes to show that partially separated cubicles, as opposed to separate rooms, are unsuited for the treatment of small-pox and chicken-pox, and of measles during the acute stage of the illness, and that there is some risk in the case of septic scarlet fever, but that scarlet fever not of a septic type, diphtheria, measles in the post eruptive stage, whooping-cough, mumps, influenza, enteric fever, and probably typhus can be treated in such a cubicle without much risk to other patients in the ward.   The resident medical officer at the Walthamstow Isolation Hospital, where the cubicles are completely separated and entered from the open air, says in 1909, " In spite of the varied nature of the cases, and the high infectivity of some of the diseases treated—such as chicken-pox and mumps—no case of infection being carried from one cubicle to another has occurred."

But whichever of the above systems may be adopted, careful nursing precautions are necessary in order to prevent cross infection if patients suffering from different diseases are attended to by the same nurse, and indeed it is claimed by some medical superintendents that with strict "aseptic" nursing patients with different infectious diseases may be safely treated in a large ward, without any physical barrier between them : see the chapter on Bed Isolation (Chapter XII).

This however postulates a high standard of training, assiduity and discipline on the part of the nursing staff, such as is not perhaps to be looked for in a small hospital where, for reasons of economy, the staff is often reduced to a minimum at a time when there are few or no patients in it, and fresh nurses are engaged from time to time as occasion requires.   Hence in such a hospital it will probably be best to provide one or more pavilions for "straightforward" cases of the prevalent diseases, and also a block containing small separate wards, approached from the open air, which will be useful under the variety of circumstances already mentioned.   The advantage claimed for the central corridor arrangement is that the work is less laborious and less trying to the nurses than in the case of compartments approached from an open verandah exposed to the inclemencies of the weather. Difficulty on this score has not however been complained of at hospitals where the latter arrangement exists.

The dimensions laid down in the Local Government Board's Memorandum for wards containing several beds are, for each bed, 12 ft. of wall space, 144 sq. ft. of floor space, and 2000 cubic ft. of air content. In order to give 2000 cubic feet, either the height of the ward must be at least 13 ft. 10½ ins. or the floor area must exceed 12 × 12 ft.; and·as a greater floor area is more useful than a greater height, the dimensions usually adopted in wards on plan C are 26 ft. width, 13 ft. height, and length = 12 ft. × half the number of beds to be provided; the beds being in two rows against the side walls.

Of the three dimensions above mentioned the most important from a medical point of view is the 12 ft. wall space, i.e. that every patient as he lies in bed shall be at least 12 ft. distant from any other patient in an adjoining bed, with a view to preventing transference of infection by contact, or by droplets of mucus expelled in coughing, etc. It is however this dimension which is apt to be encroached on during times of pressure by the placing of additional beds in the ward[1].

In single-bed wards in which each patient is effectually separated from any other, there is no advantage in a height greater than the length or breadth of the ward, and a less amount of cubic space may suffice; in the official plan D the amount is 1440 cubic ft. per bed. As regards cubic space for children Sir R. Thorne was of opinion that any reduction made in their case should be but a comparatively small one, and that the cubic space for a child should be not less than two-thirds that allowed for an adult. Dr Biernacki points out that the expulsive force exerted by a young child in coughing will not carry droplets of mucous secretion to the same distance as in the case of an adult, so that there is warrant for some reduction in the space between beds.

The Ministry of Health are now prepared to accept a floor space of 12 ft. by 10 ft. in the case of wards in a block constructed in accordance with plan D. In wards for more than a single bed the floor space per bed should be 144 superficial feet and the capacity not less than 1872 cubic feet per bed.

In the pavilions the windows should, if possible, be so spaced

---

[1] In some of the Metropolitan Asylums Board's Hospitals the wall space for diphtheria and enteric fever cases is as much as 15 ft. per bed.

in relation to the number of beds that each bed shall be between two windows and that it shall be in the line of cross-ventilation.

The best aspect for ward-blocks is with the windows on the two sides facing S.E. and N.W. as the windows then get the morning sun, and avoid it in the hottest part of the day, and avoid also the cold N.E. winds and the S.W. gales.

Verandahs on the sunny side of the wards are useful not only in an observation block for approach to the several compartments, but also in a pavilion block for purposes of open air treatment. Access to the verandah may be by a French window opening down to floor level to enable beds to be wheeled out, as at the Colne and Holme Joint Hospital. See plan in Chapter XIX.

The verandah should have a glass roof which should reach only as high as the transom of the window, leaving the uppermost light of the window free and capable of opening above the

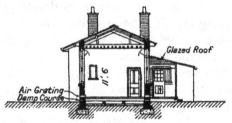

Fig. 7. Showing section of hospital building, plan B of the Local Government
Board's model.

roof (see Fig. 7 above). The verandah may have a dwarf wall in front as a screen against wind or drifting snow, but should be open between this and the roof. If in bleak situations it is deemed necessary to enclose it by a glazed front, this should be in movable panels made to turn or slide, so that it can be thrown open when desired, as on occasions when cases of different nature are under treatment in adjoining wards.

The windows of a ward should have an aggregate area, including frames, of about 1 square foot to 70 cubic feet of internal capacity of the ward, that is to between 5 and 6 square feet of floor area. If the window area falls much short of this proportion it tends to make the wards look dark and gloomy; if it is much in excess the wards are more difficult to keep warm, with the result that the ventilation is apt to be restricted.

The sill of the windows, except in the case of French windows giving access to a verandah, should be about 3 feet 6 inches above the level of the floor, and the top of the windows not more than a foot below the level of the ceiling. Sash windows are the most suitable for hospital purposes; they are often made with a board at the bottom to exclude direct draught when the lower sash is slightly raised, thus allowing air to enter in an upward direction between the upper and lower sashes. Or the Austral system may be adopted, in which there are two frames, balanced together, which turn on horizontal pivots and can be inclined at any desired angle. The upper part of the window,

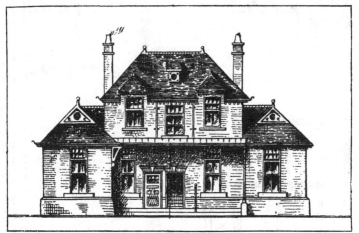

Fig. 8.   Showing elevation of a small isolation hospital, plan A of the Local
Government Board's model (see also Fig. 9, p. 94).

for about 24 inches in depth, above a transom, should be furnished with a hopper light falling inwards, and having side cheeks to prevent direct down draught.

In connection with a ward pavilion a convalescent room may be provided, where children may play or adults smoke without disturbing or inconveniencing other patients. This room may be obtained on an upper floor over the centre of the ward-block, as already mentioned, or by partitioning off the end of a long ward. Or a separate convalescent block may be erected which may be a two-storey block with day rooms on the ground floor, and dormitories on the upper floor. The air-space

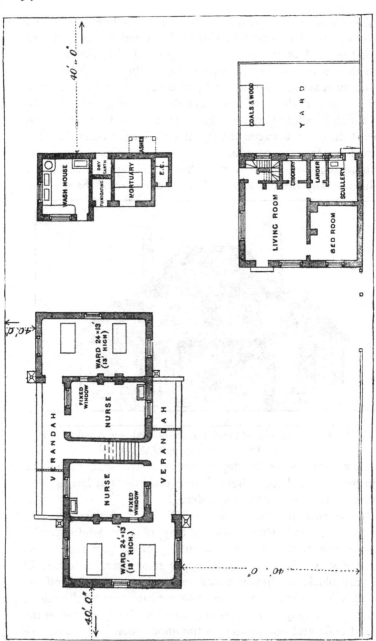

Fig. 9. Showing plan of very small hospital. (Plan A, of the Local Government Board.) Suitable for small town, village or institution. ═══ Close fence 6′ 6″ round the site.

per patient in such a block need not be so large as in a ward-block for acute cases and hence it may be erected at a smaller proportional cost. Play sheds, open at the sides, are also useful for convalescents.

Other details respecting the construction and equipment of the ward-blocks will be mentioned in the next chapter.

The out-offices will usually be one or more one-storey buildings and will comprise such places as laundry, disinfecting chamber and mortuary, and also an ambulance shed and stabling, unless local circumstances render it more convenient that the ambulance should be kept and horsed at the District Council's depôt : in this case it should be disinfected at the hospital before being sent back. Except at very small hospitals the laundry should comprise a wash house, a drying stove or closet, and an ironing room ; and in large establishments, where machinery is used, a boiler house and engine house will be necessary. The laundry should be so planned that articles which have been washed shall not come in contact with soiled ones. A foul linen receiving house, with steeping tanks for the preliminary disinfection and rinsing of infected and soiled linen, and a distributing room for finished articles, is sometimes provided, and may be useful at large hospitals. A separate staff laundry is also sometimes provided, but is hardly necessary as the staff linen can be washed on a different day from that of the patients, if their mixing is objected to.

The disinfecting chamber should contain an apparatus for the disinfection by steam of blankets, bedding and other articles which cannot be washed. There are several efficient steam disinfecting apparatus now on the market. Lyon's or the Equifex may be used at large establishments where there is a boiler, or Thresh's or the Velox which are cheaper and do not require a separate boiler, in smaller ones[1]. The disinfecting apparatus may sometimes be used for district purposes apart from the use of the hospital ; and the building in which it is

---

[1] A separate boiler is preferable where the water supply is a hard one, as the removal of the "fur" from the narrow space between the two casings, where this serves as the boiler, is a difficult matter. The life of the apparatus is shorter where it is directly exposed to the heat of the furnace than where steam is supplied from a separate boiler.

placed is often divided by a central partition into two chambers, with a door of the apparatus in each, one chamber being for the placing of articles for disinfection in the apparatus, and the other for taking them out after the process.   A small incinerator may usefully be provided for the cremation of infected rubbish and articles of clothing, etc. of small value.

For the mortuary a prominent position should be avoided, and for the sake of coolness, it should be lighted only by a north window.

In hospitals of any size a discharging block should be provided, containing an undressing room, a bathroom, and a dressing room, in which convalescents may take their final bath, and put on clean clothes before leaving the hospital.   Sometimes a room is added in which they may rest or pass a night after the bath in order to avoid the risk of catching cold by going out immediately afterwards.   The discharging rooms may adjoin the laundry block or the porter's lodge.

BIBLIOGRAPHY

Memorandum of the Local Government Board on the provision of Isolation Hospitals by Local Authorities. 1902. With Appendix. 1908.

Thorne. Hospital Report, and preface to reprint. 1901.

—— On some special arrangements for the isolation of infectious diseases. Transactions of Epidemiological Society. 1885.

Parsons. Hospital Report. 1912. With appended memoranda by B. T. Kitchin and Th. Thomson.

Nightingale, Florence. Notes on Hospitals. 1863.

Buchanan, Sir G. English Hospitals in their Sanitary Aspects. Address to Medical Society of London. 1875.

Glaister. Text-book of Public Health. Edinburgh. 1910. (Description of Victoria Hospital, Belfast, pp. 494—5), also in Journal of Sanitary Institute, Vol. xx, Pt. iv.

Caiger, F. F. Cubicle Isolation. Public Health, June, 1911.

Goodall, E. W. An account of the Isolation Chambers recently provided at the Eastern Hospital. Report of Metropolitan Asylums Board. 1910.

The Metropolitan Asylums Board of London and its Work. 1900.

Young, Meredith. Practical Hints on Isolation Hospital Construction. Public Health, Jan. 1903.

Brown, F. H. General Principles of Hospital Construction, in Buck's Hygiene and Public Health. New York, 1879. (Gives extensive bibliography.)

CHAPTER VII

DETAILS OF HOSPITAL WARD-BLOCKS

Walls. The walls of a permanent hospital are usually constructed of brick, or in districts where building stone is cheaper, of stone. The walls of the pavilions, in districts where byelaws for securing stability of walls of new buildings are in force[1], will generally be required, in view of their length and height, to be at least a brick and a half thick, and that thickness is in any case desirable for the sake of securing an equable temperature and keeping out damp. Hollow walls are useful for the same purposes, especially in exposed situations.

In a few instances hospital buildings have been constructed of the more recently introduced materials such as concrete slabs, and the Local Government Board and Ministry of Health have sanctioned loans for their erection, but further experience of their stability and durability is necessary before it can be decided how much is gained by their use[2].

There should be a damp-proof course in the walls about 6 inches above the level of the ground, and an impermeable layer of concrete or asphalte under the floors. In a few instances, as at the Huddersfield and Tolworth Hospitals, the ward-blocks have been built on arches with a view to securing dryness and ventilation under the floors, but this mode of construction is rarely necessary and adds much to the cost; it has also been found to render the wards cold. Sometimes however when a ward-block is built on sloping ground there will be a space under one end which may be utilised as a heating chamber, or covered playground for convalescents, or for storage purposes.

The walls of the wards should be lined internally with some smooth hard impermeable material which can be readily cleansed

---

[1] In the Model Byelaws of the Local Government Board as to New Buildings, temporary hospitals are exempted from the requirements of the byelaws.

[2] See as to this *Report of Departmental Committee of Board of Education on Cost of School Buildings*, 1911. Cd. 5534.

with a damp cloth.   There are various hard cements and plasters suitable for the purpose, as Keene's cement, Parian cement, selenitic plaster, etc. ; and there are materials in sheets or slabs which can be fixed to the surface, as eternite, opalite, uralite or glazed tiles.   A dado of glazed bricks is sometimes used but adds to the cost and has too many joints.

A smooth plastered surface, with distemper or lime-wash which can be renewed after use, may suffice where it is desired to keep the first cost as low as possible.

In order to avoid recesses in which dust or dirt may lodge, the corners between the walls should be rounded, and the angles between the walls and floor should be similarly rounded or filled with a wooden fillet triangular or concave in section.   In the woodwork and plastering, projections which may harbour dust should be avoided, and the mouldings should be as plain and simple as possible.   Features which involve unnecessary labour, such as bright metal fittings which have to be kept polished, should be avoided.

Floor.   The floor of the wards should be of a material that is strong, durable and not liable to crack ; it should be smooth though not slippery, impermeable and readily cleansed.   Solid floors laid down *in situ* such as cement, terrazzo, papyrolith, asbolith and doloment are impermeable so long as they are in sound condition, but they are liable to crack through settling of the ground, or through the shrinking that occurs in the neighbourhood of a stove or over the course of hot water pipes.   Some such materials contain sawdust and are liable to get rough through wear.   Hard floors as cement and terrazzo are sometimes complained of as cold and tiring to the feet.

If a wooden floor is preferred great care should be taken to obtain well-seasoned wood which will not shrink.   Through shrinking wooden blocks become loose, and cracks form between the boards of a boarded floor in which dirt may lodge and through which foul liquids may gain access to the space under the floor.   A well-laid floor of oak, pitch-pine or teak, polished with beeswax and turpentine, melted paraffin wax or "Ronuk" is durable, impervious and readily cleansed, but is expensive, and its slipperiness is an objection.   Probably an ordinary boarded floor tongued and grooved is sufficiently satisfactory if covered with linoleum or other suitable impermeable floor cloth. The floor cloth should be of good quality and thickness, with as few joints as possible, the edges being carefully fitted and fastened down.

Ceiling. The wards should be ceiled under the roof, with a view to protection against heat and cold. If the wards extend partly into the roof, there should be a ceiling under any timbers or tie-rods upon which infectious dust might lodge.

Ventilation. Natural ventilation by windows and ventilating openings is relied on in hospital wards, unless under exceptional circumstances such as at the Victoria Hospital, Belfast, and the compartments at the Eastern Hospital already mentioned. The points to be observed in the construction of windows have been set out in the last chapter. In addition to the windows, inlets under the beds, with provision for breaking up the entering current of air so as to avoid draughts, and Tobin tubes in the walls are often provided, and sometimes ventilating shafts and cowls in the roof. Ventilating stoves admitting warmed fresh air are useful. An extraction shaft may be placed in the roof surrounding the stove pipe, or adjoining a chimney flue.

Warming. Care should be taken to provide the wards with ample means of warming; not unfrequently the means originally provided have been found insufficient. This care is especially necessary where the hospital is on a cold and bleak site, and where the wards have much outside wall in proportion to their capacity, or a large area of glass. In small wards, of 1 to 4 beds, an ordinary fireplace in the wall is sufficient; but in larger wards the question will arise whether the heating will be best effected by stoves or open fireplaces; by a system of hot water pipes; or by both methods combined.

Open fireplaces have a cheerful appearance and give a pleasanter heat than hot water pipes; the heat being given off in the radiant form, whereas the heating from hot water pipes is mainly effected by convection of warmed air. Warming by hot water pipes involves less labour to the nurses, and is more effective and uniform and more economical than that by fireplaces, especially where the amount of elevation of temperature required is a large one, as on a cold site. In such a situation the two methods may be combined, a pipe-heating system being adopted, together with fireplaces in reduced number, for the purposes of cheerfulness, ventilation and radiant heat.

Where more than one fireplace is required owing to the length of the ward, the fireplaces should be placed so as to give as uniform a distribution of heat as possible. There may be one in each end wall, or one in each side wall, placed alternately, not opposite to one another; or there may be a central double-faced open stove. Central stoves are often made, as in Shorland's and Musgrave's, with descending flues which pass under the floor to a chimney at the side of the ward. This arrangement has the advantage that there is no obstruction to the view across the ward, but upright flues are now made of glazed pottery, which are ornamental and block the view much less than the brick stacks formerly used. On the other hand stoves with descending flues are more costly, and are liable to go wrong and smoke, and the heat from the underground horizontal flue is apt to cause shrinking and cracking of the floor as already mentioned. To avoid smoking the effective height of the flue, i.e. its length above the level of the fireplace, should be at least twice the length of the horizontal portion. In the lower wards of two-storey blocks, where a high chimney can be obtained, stoves with descending flues are convenient and generally act well. Closed stoves are more economical of fuel than open grates, but do not assist ventilation in the same degree or afford so pleasant a heat, and the flue is apt to get overheated and give off noxious fumes, iron being somewhat pervious to carbon monoxide at a high temperature.

In a system of heating by hot water, the heating coils—usually called "radiators," though inappropriately, as they heat the room by convection of hot air rather than by radiation—are best placed and distributed along the sides of the ward, under windows. There may be a ventilating inlet near the floor behind each coil so that the incoming air may be warmed. In a low-pressure system there should be 12 ft. of hot water piping for every 1000 cubic feet of air to be warmed. Heating coils should also be placed in the bathrooms and sanitary annexes in order to protect the water pipes from freezing. In a high-pressure system there is a closed circuit of strong wrought iron pipes, in which water can be heated to a temperature of 300° F., whereas in a low-pressure system the temperature attainable falls short of the boiling point, 212° F. In a high-pressure system therefore the pipes are smaller, and the length of piping required is less, 8 or 9 feet being required for every 1000 cubic feet of space to be warmed. The pipes should be protected in order to prevent persons coming into contact with them, as owing to their high temperature a severe burn can be inflicted.

Similar remarks apply to a system of heating by pipes in which steam circulates. In this case arrangements are necessary for the return of condensed water to the boiler.

Where the heating of a ward is effected by a system of hot pipes, or by closed stoves, the air is apt to be dried to an unpleasant degree; in such cases evaporating vessels should be provided and kept filled with water, so as to maintain the air at a more suitable degree of moisture.

The water in a hot water system may be heated either by a boiler (or furnace in the case of a high-pressure system, in which there is no separate boiler) for each individual block, or by a central boiler for all the blocks, or, where a supply of steam is available, by steam through a calorifier. The choice of the method of warming will depend in a measure on the arrangement and use of the hospital and on the amount of heating required. If the buildings are compactly and conveniently arranged on the site and if several of them are commonly in use at a time, there will be a saving of fuel and labour in heating from a central furnace, instead of from separate furnaces for each block or from a number of fireplaces. On the other hand if the ward-blocks are small and scattered, the length of piping required and the loss of heat in distribution will be proportionally large; and the saving in current expenditure effected by heating from a central furnace may probably not counterbalance the interest on the capital cost. Also if many of the ward-blocks are often empty, separate furnaces may be preferable on the ground that it is wasteful to have to keep a large boiler heated when only a small amount of work has to be done; complicated installations too are apt to get out of order and deteriorate when not in use. For these reasons in very small hospitals and in those which, like small-pox hospitals, may only rarely be in use, open fireplaces or stoves will probably be preferable to more elaborate methods.

In large hospitals a system of steam distribution from a central boiler or boilers (which should be in duplicate) has many advantages as, for example, for purposes of furnishing a supply of hot water, heating sterilisers, and feeding jets for inhalation in throat cases.

For details of methods of heating the reader is referred to treatises on Warming and Ventilation.

Hot Water supply. An ample supply of hot water is required in hospitals for baths and for various washing purposes, and care should be taken to provide it as the arrangements originally made for the purpose have often in practice proved to be insufficient.

Where there is a supply of steam from a central boiler, a calorifier, heated by steam, may be used for the supply of hot water to baths; or in other cases, a special boiler may be provided for the purpose in a chamber in the basement. It is not advisable to draw off hot water from the circulating pipes used for warming. In small blocks hot water is usually obtained from a cylinder, the water being heated by a boiler connected with the fireplace in the nurses' duty room; but such a cylinder will not afford a supply sufficient for many baths at a time. Where gas is available a geyser may be used for furnishing a supply of hot water, but the danger of using such an apparatus without a flue to carry off the poisonous products of combustion should be borne in mind, and careful supervision is necessary.

Bath Rooms. One bathroom may conveniently serve for a ward-block of about 12 beds, sometimes even 16, and it is usually placed in the centre portion of the block, so as to be near to both wards and to the duty room from which the supply of hot water is obtained, as in the official plan C[1].

---

[1] See Fig. 1, p. 81.

Where the number of beds in a ward exceeds 12 it is desirable that the ward should have a separate bathroom approached direct from it ; and this may be either in the centre of the block or in an annexe at the end or side of the ward.

Movable baths are sometimes provided, especially where one bath has to serve for several small wards, but nurses usually find the labour of wheeling to the ward a bath full of water, with the risk of its slopping over, greater than that of taking a patient to the bathroom or of "blanket-bathing" in the ward. The liability to slop over may be obviated by the upper edge of the bath being made to bend over inwards.

For convenience in use and economy of hot water the baths should not be too deep and should have sloping sides and rounded bottoms, not flat bottoms with a seam in which dirt may lodge where the bottom meets the sides. For the use of children additional small baths, requiring less water, may advantageously be provided, and these should be fixed on a raised base, or if movable, on legs, so as to involve less stooping for the nurses.

Sanitary annexes. The water closets and slop sinks, as already mentioned, should be placed in annexes separated from the wards by cross-ventilated lobbies. The usual position of the annexe is at the end of the ward, but in the case of very long wards it is more convenient of access if placed at the side. In large wards a second water closet may be necessary, and may conveniently be of a size suitable for children. A separate closet for the nurses is sometimes provided.

The water closets in hospitals are now always of the bracket or pedestal form and usually on the "wash down" principle. The seat is hinged, and may conveniently be made wider than the pan, so that feeble patients may be able to raise themselves by resting their hands on it, or handrails may be fixed in the side walls for the same purpose.

The slop sink should be placed in a closet in the same annexe ; it should be of a kind suitable to receive slop water and contents of bed-pans—not an ordinary kitchen sink—with a 3-inch waste pipe not discharging over a gulley but ventilated like a soil pipe. Water taps supplied with hot and cold water and suitable for the cleansing of bed-pans and other vessels, should be placed over the sink, and it should have a sloping enamelled ledge for draining such utensils. Shelves should also be fixed for storing them. A small ordinary kitchen sink should also be provided.

Slop sinks of suitable patterns may be obtained from the makers of sanitary ware.

Where aseptic nursing is adopted a steriliser will find its place in the sanitary annexes.

There may also be a lavatory basin, and an opening in the wall through which soiled linen may be put into a vessel containing a disinfectant solution for removal to the laundry without carrying it through the wards.

Drainage. The drains should be constructed and ventilated on the usual principles, and the drains of each ward-block should be connected to the common drain in the way that those of separate houses are connected to a sewer. Where the sewage has to be treated on the site it will generally be advisable to provide separate means of disposal for the roof water, and if the water supply of the hospital is hard, the rainwater may with advantage be stored for washing purposes.

Furniture. The furniture of an isolation hospital ward should be strong, simple in pattern, and of a kind to be easily kept clean. There are on the market bedsteads, chairs, bedstands and tables of white enamelled metal which are well designed and not expensive. Cumbering the ward with superfluous articles should be avoided.

Artificial Lighting. If the hospital site is within reach of mains for the supply of electric current or gas, the most convenient and economical means of lighting will be to have a supply of one or the other laid on. Electric lighting has the well-known advantages of not adding undesirable products of combustion to the air, nor blackening the ceilings, etc., and of convenience in use; but the corresponding disadvantages of gas are much less in the case of modern incandescent burners than with the old flat flame; and gas, besides being cheaper, is useful as a source of heat, for cooking, heating water for baths, etc. When used for heating purposes, however, there should always be a flue to carry off the products of combustion, as a poisonous gas, carbon monoxide, is liable to be formed when a flame impinges on a cooler body.

Where a public service of electricity or gas is not available, the question may arise of providing a supply by a private installation. At a large institution this may be advisable, but at a small hospital or at one which, like a small-pox hospital, may be unoccupied for long periods, it will probably be not worth the cost. Acetylene gas has been used occasionally at isolation hospitals, but has not always been found satisfactory. The generating house should be a detached building, and the need for precautions in the storage of calcium carbide must be remembered.

At small hospitals where gas or electricity is not available the usual means of lighting is by lamps burning mineral oil. "Petrolite" lamps, burning petrol vapour with incandescent mantles, give a good light. All such arrangements involve the need of caution against fire.

BIBLIOGRAPHY

Memorandum of the Local Government Board on the provision of Isolation Hospitals by Local Authorities. 1902.

Thorne. Hospital Report, and preface to reprint. 1901.

Parsons. Hospital Report, 1912, and appended memorandum by B. T. Kitchin.

Report of Departmental Committee on Cost of School Buildings, Board of Education. 1911. [Cd. 5534.]

Nightingale, Florence. Notes on Hospitals. 1863.

Glaister. Text-book of Public Health. 1910.

Young, Meredith. Practical Hints on Isolation Hospital Construction. Public Health, Jan. 1903.

Brown in Buck's Hygiene and Public Health. 1879.

Jones, Herbert. Notes on a few points of detail in the construction of Isolation Hospitals. Public Health, May, 1897.

Shaw, W. N., F.R.S. Article on Ventilation and Warming in Stevenson's Hygiene.

CHAPTER VIII

MOVABLE HOSPITALS AND HOSPITALS OF MORE OR LESS PERISHABLE CONSTRUCTION

It has been already mentioned that in many districts the first attempts at the isolation of infectious diseases were made during epidemics, either in existing buildings, rarely suitable for the purpose, or in temporary buildings hurriedly erected. On the conclusion of the epidemic, this emergency hospital has sometimes been given up ; in other instances it has continued in existence, but has in practice been little, if at all, used ; in others again recognition of the usefulness of isolation has led to the erection of permanent hospital accommodation, in connection with which the temporary building, if suitable, may have been utilised. This chapter does not deal with the improvising in an emergency of "temporary places for the reception of the sick"—as to which see Chapter III—but with means for supplementing during an epidemic the accommodation afforded by a permanent hospital, and with structures of sufficient durability to be of service when the emergency is over.

I.   Portable structures capable of being rapidly erected.

In the presence of an epidemic, tents or huts are sometimes useful as a means of temporary extension of an existing hospital, if space for their erection exists on the site, and they can be administered from it. Tents however are not suitable in very cold, wet or rough weather. The following remarks as to hospital tents are taken from a Memorandum by the Medical Officer of the Local Government Board in 1876 :

"As to Tents. It is essential to secure the dryness of the ground upon which they are pitched by trenching around and between them, so as to carry off all rainfall and prevent the lodgment of moisture. The tents should everywhere be distant at least a diameter and a half from each other. The approaches should be paved or otherwise prepared, to prevent their being trodden into mud in wet weather, and it is especially requisite that abundant proper means be provided for the reception of refuse matter, and that no casting of slops or other refuse upon the ground in the vicinity of the tents be allowed. In the distribution of patients in the active stages of the disease not more than one patient should be assigned to a bell tent of the ordinary regulation size, nor more than three such patients to the regulation hospital marquee; and in other forms of tents the number of patients should be regulated in similar proportions." [Size of regulation bell tent: Diameter, 14 ft.; height, 10 ft.; area of base, 154 sq. ft.; cubic space, 513 ft. Size of regulation hospital marquee: Length, 29 ft.; width, 14 ft.; side walls, 5 ft. 4 in.;

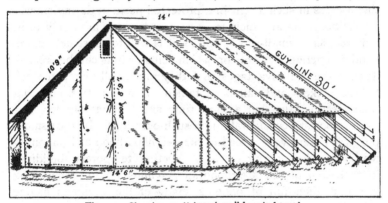

Fig. 10. Showing an "American" hospital tent[1].

height to ridge, 11 ft. 8 in.; area of base, 396 sq. ft.; cubic space, 3366 ft.]

"Tents should always be provided with special ventilating openings. They should have boarded floors raised sufficiently above the ground, so as to allow of air passing freely beneath. From the ready inflammability of the ordinary canvas of which tents are constructed, much care is required in the use of lights in tents, and tents should not be used in states of weather which render artificial warming necessary, if sufficiently rapid provision for the isolation of the sick can otherwise be had. The safest method of warming a hospital marquee is by a flue carried beneath the floor from a stove placed in an excavation outside the tent to a chimney also beyond the tent wall."

[1] Reproduced from a sketch kindly lent by Dr J. S. Tew.

Dr Tew, medical officer of health of Tonbridge, has used successfully in emergencies as an adjunct to permanent hospitals the "American" hospital tent, made by Edgington, 2 Duke St., London Bridge, which measures 14 ft. 6 in. × 14 ft., and costs £14[1]. The tents can be placed end to end and latched together so as to make a ward of any required length. The roof is of two layers of canvas, but as these come very close together in the upper part, it is an improvement to put up a second cross pole, so as to keep them parallel. The tent is warmed by a "tortoise" slow combustion stove, the pipe as it passes through a hole in the canvas being protected by asbestos. He has treated diphtheria cases in such a tent in a protected position during snow.

At hospitals at which temporary extensions are likely to be required, as at small-pox hospitals, it is well to construct beforehand a concrete platform on which tents or huts can be erected. Tents have the advantages that they are usually kept in stock by the makers and can be obtained at short notice, and that their erection takes but a short time and requires but few men —an important consideration on such occasions. In 1901 small-pox was extensively spread in the neighbourhood of London by workmen who contracted it in erecting temporary buildings in extension of the Metropolitan Asylums Board's Small-Pox Hospital, then full of patients, many of the workmen having refused re-vaccination. See Chapter IX.

It has been suggested that the rapid extension (temporary) of small-pox hospitals can best be effected by having platforms, on concrete, constructed at each site on which standard size sectional buildings of timber construction can be rapidly put up. If a single authority in each county was responsible for the isolation of small-pox, one stock standard size for all institutions could be sent out with all necessary fittings and furniture and erected as occasion required ; this would economise expenditure for superfluous temporary buildings that would become necessary if each district had to provide for its own emergencies. A pavilion could be constructed on the sectional system in a few days, probably in a week at most from the time the sections and fittings etc. were on the site. It is possible that the use of temporary sectional

---

[1] See Fig. 10 on p. 107.

camp buildings, not now required by the military since the conclusion of the war, might be largely adopted for the above purpose.

Berthon Huts. The Berthon hut or tent[1], made by the Berthon Boat Co., Romsey, Hampshire, is a dome-shaped polygonal structure of wood, made in segments so that it can be easily taken to pieces and put together. It has a wooden floor stained and varnished. The roof is made of timbers radiating from the apex, between which are stretched two layers of canvas made waterproof with flexible paint. The walls are of two thicknesses

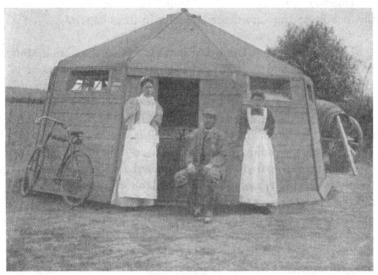

Fig. 11.   Berthon Hut, in use as a temporary hospital by Sevenoaks Rural District Council.   From a photograph by Dr J. S. Tew.

of match-board, with glass windows in each segment. Ventilation is by fresh air entering between the double sides, and escaping by ventilators at the apex. Warming is by a slow combustion stove in the centre, with a stove pipe projecting through the apex nowhere touching any wood or canvas. The canvas is said to be hard to ignite, and when ignited only smoulders away slowly. The price of a hospital hut 18 ft. in diameter is £50.

Dr J. S. Tew states in a letter that in the Sevenoaks Rural District two of these huts are kept stored in case of small-pox

[1] See illustration above.

occurring, and he has found them fairly satisfactory, but it was very difficult to keep up the temperature in cold weather without closing up windows so that ventilation became inadequate. They withstood the weather well if kept in very good repair, but after a hot spell, followed by rain, warping of the wood often took place with consequent leakage. They were useful as an adjunct, where there was administrative accommodation available, but one of them used as a kitchen was inconvenient. Storage for long periods was detrimental, and repairs were generally required before re-erection.

Doecker hospitals of the "light" construction come under this heading; they are described later in this chapter.

II. Hospitals constructed of materials other than brick, stone or similar substances, are commonly spoken of as "temporary," although with care and under favourable circumstances they may last for a number of years. They were not usually regarded by the late Local Government Board as "permanent works" suitable to be paid for by means of loan. The Board said:

"Temporary buildings, as, for instance, buildings constructed of wood or corrugated iron, are ill suited for permanent use as hospitals, for the reason that it is difficult to maintain them at a proper temperature during extremes of hot and cold weather; moreover they are less durable than brick or stone buildings, requiring more frequent repairs in order to keep them in a properly weather-proof condition, and they are liable to be destroyed by fire and storm. *It is not the practice of the Local Government Board in ordinary cases to sanction loans for iron hospitals or for hospital buildings of temporary character.*"

Short loans have, however, been sanctioned for such buildings in exceptional cases, as for instance for extension, during an epidemic, of an approved permanent hospital, and the Board are willing to sanction, in connection with proposals to erect hospitals of this kind, loans for purchase of site, fencing, drainage, water supply, furniture, and other works which would be of value towards the ultimate erection of a permanent hospital, and also for brick foundations, if so planned as to be suitable for the subsequent erection on them of a permanent building complying with the Board's usual requirements. The hospitals which are sold ready-made by makers do not however usually comply with these requirements, being deficient in space per bed, administrative accommodation and other respects.

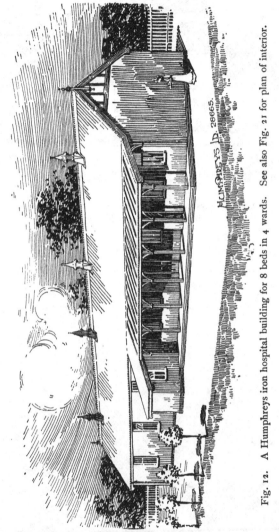

Fig. 12.   A Humphreys iron hospital building for 8 beds in 4 wards.   See also Fig. 21 for plan of interior.

The annexed figures, 12 to 23, for which the author is indebted to Messrs Humphreys, of Knightsbridge, London[1],

[1] Similar hospitals are made by Speirs & Co., Glasgow, and have been largely used in Scotland.

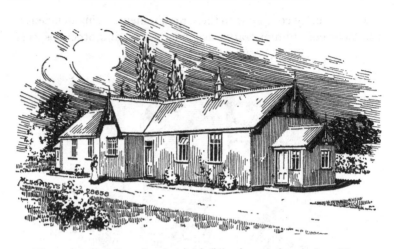

Fig. 13.   A Humphreys iron hospital building for 12 beds.   A plan of the interior is shown in Fig. 19.

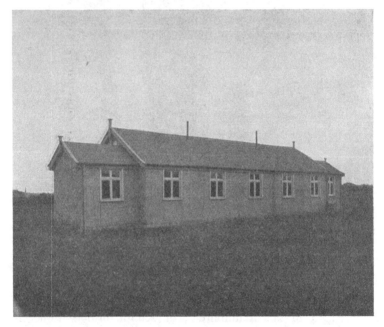

Fig. 14.   Another form of a Humphreys iron hospital building for 12 beds. For plan see Fig. 17.

illustrate some of the forms of iron and other hospitals made by them.

Messrs Humphreys's hospitals are made in the following types:

1. Standard type. Walls and roofs of standard pattern galvanized corrugated iron, with internal lining of varnished match-boarding.

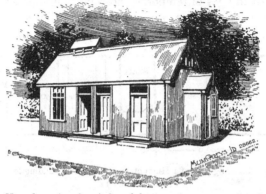

Fig. 15.   Humphreys iron hospital wash-house and mortuary. See also Fig. 23.

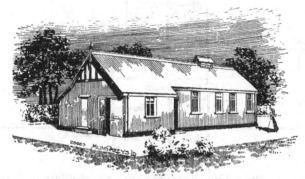

Fig. 16.   Humphreys iron hospital laundry, ambulance, etc. See also Fig. 22.

2. A more pleasing appearance is obtained by the use of Italian sheeting to the roofs.

3. The walls of the buildings are frequently overlaid with timber bands, producing the effect of old-fashioned half-timbered structures.

4. Walls of plain corrugated iron ; roofs of asbestos-cement, lozenge-shaped tiles, red, white or grey colour.

P.   8

5. Walls of asbestos-cement fireproof sheeting; roofs of asbestos-cement, red, white or grey colour.

6. Internal lining of asbestos-cement fireproof sheeting in lieu of match-boarding.

7. Walls in rough cast plaster, and roofs in asbestos-cement tiles, Broseley tiles, or reed-thatching.

The advantages of temporary hospital buildings are:

1. They can be erected in less time than a permanent building, and are thus useful in an emergency, such as an epidemic.

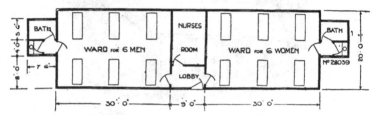

Fig. 17. Showing plan of a Humphreys iron hospital building for 12 beds. See also Fig. 14.

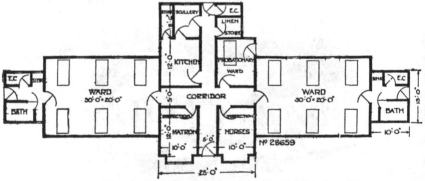

Fig. 18. Plan of a Humphreys iron hospital with administrative offices.

It has often happened, however, that when the erection of a hospital has been deferred until an epidemic was present, even a temporary hospital has not been able to be got ready before the epidemic has come to an end, or at any rate before the time when it would have been most useful has passed.

2. The need for a hospital may be only temporary, as for instance for the use of a colony of navvies engaged upon a large

engineering work, such as waterworks or a long tunnel, in a sparsely populated district, who will be dispersed when the work is completed, or in a district dependent on a colliery which is approaching exhaustion.

3. The cost is less than that of a building of brick or stone and may thus be within the means of a small district which could not afford to erect a permanent hospital.

The apparent cheapness is, however, to a considerable extent illusory. It must be remembered that the maker's list price includes only the bare building; site, fencing, water supply, drainage, foundations, concrete under floor, furniture and fittings, are all extras, and thus it has happened that an iron hospital of which the catalogue price was £400 has come to cost more than

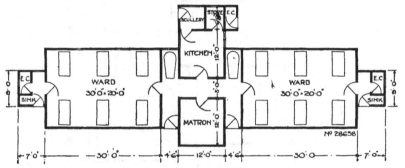

Fig. 19. Plan of a Humphreys hospital building, for elevation of which see Fig. 13.

£1000 before it was completed. The accommodation moreover in such a hospital is usually suitable for only one disease at a time, the space per bed is scanty and the administrative accommodation at a minimum.

These deficiencies however will not so much matter if the building is to be erected in extension of an existing hospital, or on a site on which there is already a house which will serve for the accommodation of the staff.

The ready-made hospital buildings sold by makers usually consist of a timber framework covered externally with corrugated iron, weather-boarding or some proprietary material, and lined internally with match-boarding, with a wooden floor. Those erected locally have sometimes been covered with boards and roofed with

8—2

tarred felt, "wire-wove," or other material. The defects of these buildings are largely due to the match-board lining, in spite of its cheerful appearance when new and freshly varnished. It gets very dry and highly inflammable, and as the flame readily runs along

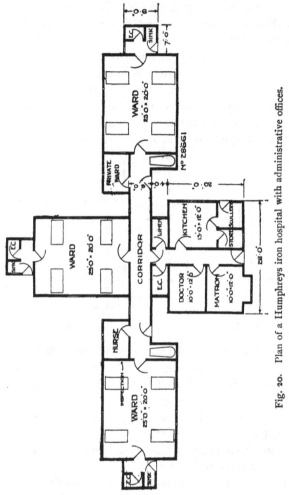

Fig. 20.   Plan of a Humphreys iron hospital with administrative offices.

the spaces between the timbers, buildings of this sort have in many instances been rapidly consumed, in some cases with loss of life. The especial point of danger is where the flue of the stove passes through the roof or wall. Owing to the difficulty of keeping up the temperature in cold weather in such buildings, a large fire is made and the stove pipe gets overheated. Other objections are that the crevices of the boarding afford lodgment for dirt and vermin and

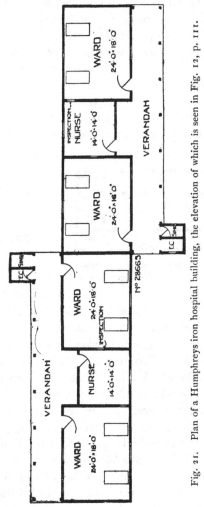

Fig. 21.   Plan of a Humphreys iron hospital building, the elevation of which is seen in Fig. 12, p. 111.

render efficient disinfection difficult, and that they gape when the boards shrink and allow cold draughts to come through into the ward. These objections to timber-frame buildings are, however, lessened when they are lined internally with lath and plaster or

with some impermeable and fireproof material in sheets, but it is
said that this takes longer to put up and increases the cost.

Frame buildings covered with wood or iron have also been on
several occasions blown over or wrecked during a storm, causing
much hardship to the patients; and they are hot in summer,
cold in winter and noisy in hail storms or heavy rain.

The duration of frame buildings covered with wood or corrugated iron will depend partly on the original strength and quality
of the materials and on the manner in which they were put
together, and partly on the care taken of the buildings and the
execution of repairs when required. With care such a building
on brick foundations may last (barring accidents) 15 or even 20

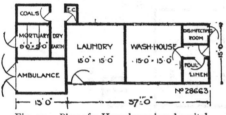

Fig. 22.   Plan of a Humphreys iron hospital
laundry, ambulance, etc. For elevation see
Fig. 16.

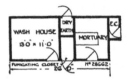

Fig. 23. Plan of a Humphreys
hospital wash-house and
mortuary; see also Fig. 15.

years, but frequent repairs will be needed in the later years in
order to keep it in a habitable condition.

Doecker Hospitals. The "Doecker" system of construction of
portable buildings was invented many years ago by Captain von
Doecker of the Danish Army, but has since been improved from
time to time[1]. Doecker buildings have been largely used on the
continent as hospitals, and have recently come into use in this
country for the purposes of elementary schools. The present
agents in this country are the Hygienic Constructions and Portable
Buildings Co., Limited, Stockholm Road, South Bermondsey.
There are two modes of construction, the "Strong" and the "Light."
The former is intended to form a substitute for substantial buildings
of brick or stone, and the latter is intended for temporary pur-

[1] The term "Doecker hospital" appears during the past 25 years to have been
sometimes loosely used in this country as a general term for portable hospital buildings,
not necessarily of Doecker construction. The "Ducker" hospital, made by an American
firm, is a wooden frame building, without any special features calling for description here.

poses, where frequent removal may be required, and portability, rapidity of erection and small cost are the main desiderata.

In both constructions the buildings are made in sections, each about 3 ft. 3 in. wide, which are fastened together with iron hooks and studs; this method enables the building to be taken to pieces and altered in form or re-erected elsewhere.

In the "Strong construction" the sections are of stout timber frames covered on the outside with morticed weather-boards and on the inside with sheets of a composition called the "Doecker material," which, it is claimed, is non-inflammable and water- and acid-proof. Between the outer and inner walls is a cavity which is divided by layers of insulating material with a view to afford a better protection against external heat or cold. The total thickness of the wall is about $4\frac{1}{2}$ inches. In a building of this construction exhibited at the International Conference on School Hygiene in 1907, the principals of the roof were latticed wrought-iron girders, with iron tie-rods, and were supported by iron pillars resting on piers of brickwork. The fastenings of the sections were concealed by wooden fillets nailed or screwed over them and painted. This would rather take away from the readiness with which the building could be taken to pieces and put together again. The floor was of wood with a ventilated space beneath it, and was covered with linoleum.

The roof is usually of double boarding with an air space between, and is covered with a flexible and water-proof material ("ruberoyd"); or there may be a single thickness of boarding, with a ceiling under the roof, which is preferable. The stove pipe is carried through the roof in an outer tube, the space between the two tubes being packed with a non-conducting material as a precaution against fire. It is claimed that hospitals of this construction will last with care 30—40 years or more.

In the "Light construction" the wooden framework is lighter, and is covered with sheets of Doecker material on both sides. The whole building, including walls, flooring and roof, is in sections, and the floor is so constructed that it forms packing covers for the remainder of the building, thus saving weight, space, and freight in transit. No foundation is required, as the building rests on wooden feet, which can be adjusted to inequalities of the ground. Buildings of this construction are made of a standard size, 50 × 16 ft., which is often kept in stock, and a building of this kind can be erected complete in one day by unskilled labour. The price, without internal partitions, is £237. When not required for use, it can be taken down and stored.

Portable hospitals of this construction were used by the German Red Cross Society during the cold of a Manchurian winter in the Russo-Japanese war, and they have also been used in the tropical heat of South-West Africa.

For other illustrations of buildings of materials other than brick or stone see the chapter on Sanatoria, Chapter XVIII.

BIBLIOGRAPHY

Thorne. Hospital Report, 1882, with appended Memorandum of the Local Government Board on Hospitals of 1876.

Parsons. Hospital Report. 1912.

Memorandum of the Local Government Board on the construction and arrangement of inexpensive buildings for tuberculous patients, 1913.

Gold, D. D. The control and isolation of infectious diseases in thinly populated counties. Public Health, May 1912.

CHAPTER IX

SMALL-POX HOSPITALS

IT has long been recognised that small-pox stands in a different category from the other infectious diseases, and requires to be treated apart from them. In London the first small-pox hospital, as we have seen, was established in 1746, while the London Fever Hospital was not started until 1802[1].

Dr Bristowe and Mr T. Holmes at their inquiry in 1863

---

[1] The London Small-Pox Hospital was first established at King's Cross, then in the country, but in 1815 the building was occupied by the London Fever Hospital, which, when the ground was required by the Great Northern Railway in 1848, was removed to Islington. The Small-Pox Hospital was re-established about the same time at Highgate, on a site then free from surrounding buildings, but in 1896 the neighbourhood having then become populous, it was removed to Clare Hall, near Barnet. It had hitherto been on a charitable basis, but in 1907 it was taken over by a Joint Hospital Board for the use of a number of districts in Middlesex.

found that there were very few general hospitals at which cases of small-pox were admitted, even into a detached building, and they did not recommend that they should be treated in general wards, though they recommended that typhus cases should be so treated.

The special characters of small-pox distinguishing it from other infectious diseases are its loathsome, dangerous and disfiguring nature, which renders it justly an object of dread, so that when it occurs public opinion will sanction for its prevention measures more drastic and expenditure greater than for that of the ordinary infectious diseases. It is highly infectious, and the contagium readily attaches itself to fomites, and long retains its virulence, as shown by outbreaks among workpeople handling rags at paper-mills, or cotton imported from countries where small-pox was prevalent. Small-pox has a much longer " striking distance " than any other infectious disease, and whether or not we accept the opinion that the contagium is capable of being wafted for long distances through the air, there is no doubt that small-pox tends to spread around hospitals in which cases are under treatment in a way that other infectious diseases do not[1]. For this reason it is necessary that small-pox should not be treated at the same hospital with other diseases, even in a separate block, but in a special hospital in an isolated situation.

On the other hand there are circumstances which render the results of hospital isolation in the case of small-pox far more satisfactory than in that of other infectious diseases. We have already mentioned how the dread which it inspires renders sanitary authorities and the public willing to take and submit to measures for its prevention beyond what they would for that of any other indigenous infectious disease. Small-pox patients bear removal well, and a distance of 20 or 30 miles does not prevent their being taken to hospital in a suitable ambulance. It is possible also by means of vaccination and re-vaccination to surround the patient with a cordon of immune persons. The disease,

[1] Sir Thomas Watson in his lectures (1838) says, " There is no contagion so strong and sure as that of small-pox ; none that operates at so great a distance," and these words accord with the present state of knowledge.

moreover, runs a definite course, leaving the patient, if he recovers, almost completely protected against another attack and without liability to the prolonged or recurrent infectiveness which causes so much difficulty with scarlet fever and diphtheria[1]. The disease may get a footing through the nature of the first cases being overlooked—and this is liable to happen both with the mild cases which may be mistaken for chicken-pox, and with the virulent and highly infective hæmorrhagic cases which are fatal before the characteristic rash is evident—and the infection may attach itself to the clothes or bodies of healthy persons and be passively carried by them; it does not, however, propagate itself in such positions but in due time dies out, so that such persons, once cleansed from external infection, do not remain active carriers. Hence it comes about that under modern methods of sanitary administration, small-pox in this country now frequently entirely dies out, and a large city or county may be wholly free from the disease for months or even years together until it is introduced from an outside source, as, for instance, at a seaport by a seaman from some country where small-pox is prevalent; by a tramp, or other wanderer, sojourning at a common lodging-house or casual ward; or by infected rags at a paper-mill. It results from the foregoing considerations that though the usefulness of small-pox hospitals (if properly situated) is unquestionable, they may be void of patients for long periods together; that there is especial advantage in combination of districts for the provision of small-pox hospitals, whereby the cost to any individual district of maintenance of the hospital when empty may be diminished, and that such a combination may conveniently embrace a larger number of districts and a wider area than a combination for hospital provision for other infectious diseases. Small-pox should not be treated in a hospital in a populous situation nor in one in which cases

---

[1] Dr D. S. Davies (*loc. cit.*) says, " The causal organism of small-pox is highly selective in regard to the soil on which it grows and will grow neither on an unsuitable nor on an exhausted soil. If the soil is unsuitable, the person exposed to infection neither contracts small-pox nor carries it; the infection simply dies out. If the soil is suitable the disease runs its acute course; after which the soil becomes exhausted, and the disease cannot and never does persist in the patient. So we get no chronic cases and no return cases."

of other infectious diseases are treated at the same time. The accommodation in the small-pox hospital may, however, be utilised at times when the disease is absent, as a convalescent hospital for scarlet fever or diphtheria patients, or as a sanatorium for cases of pulmonary tuberculosis. For these purposes, a position in the open country, such as is required for a small-pox hospital, is favourable. If, however, the hospital is put to such a use arrangements should be planned beforehand by which it can be cleared of other patients at short notice in the event of small-pox occurring or threatening, otherwise the district will be left without the protection which the hospital has been founded to afford.

Assuming that the hospital will be in the main reserved for small-pox, the circumstance that it will probably be for long periods without patients should be borne in mind in planning it. It will be a reason for keeping the capital cost as low as possible consistently with reasonable efficiency. In a building to be permanently and constantly occupied it may be ultimate economy to have the best and most substantial construction and equipment; but in a building which will be unused for much of the time cheaper methods may suffice. Similarly labour-saving appliances which will save their cost in a building constantly in use, are less likely to do so in one only occasionally used, and rarely to its full capacity. Ornament and luxury are out of place in such a building. The amount of accommodation to be provided need not be so great as might conceivably be required on the occasion of an epidemic; there should be a nucleus of permanent accommodation in constant readiness, with facilities for rapid extension if need should arise.

It is often difficult for reasons already mentioned in Chapter V to obtain a suitable and conveniently central site for a small-pox hospital, the proximity of such an establishment being not unnaturally objected to. The fact that it may serve a wide area gives, however, a greater choice of locality. An existing house of a convenient size to serve as an administration block, with ground on which ward-blocks may be erected, *e.g.* a small isolated farmstead, may sometimes be purchased.

The limits of population in the neighbourhood of the site,

prescribed by the late Local Government Board (and continued by the Ministry of Health) in the case of small-pox hospitals for which their sanction is required, have been already mentioned. They are:

1st. The site must not have within a quarter of a mile of it either a hospital whether for infectious diseases or not, or a workhouse, asylum, or any similar establishment, or a population of as many as 200 persons.

2nd. The site must not have within half a mile of it as many as 600 persons, whether in one or more institutions, or in dwelling-houses.

3rd. Even where the above conditions are fulfilled a hospital must not be used at one and the same time for the reception of cases of small-pox and of any other class of disease.

These limitations do not, of course, remove any danger from the hospital to persons who live within the distances mentioned from it ; but where the number of such persons is limited it will be easier to keep them under observation and see to their vaccination, and the opportunities for the spread of infection will be fewer.

A site sufficiently isolated to be suitable for a small-pox hospital will often be beyond reach of sewers and water-mains, and will have to be provided with means of sewage disposal and water supply of its own. But no danger to health arises from the admission of the sewage from a small-pox hospital into public sewers[1], and where such a method of disposal is practicable it should be adopted. In planning disposal works regard may be had to the circumstance that the volume of sewage may at times be very small, if any, and that the land may have long periods of rest.

A water supply on the premises should be provided if possible. At some temporary small-pox hospitals water has had to be brought by carting, but this, besides the expense, is undesirable as multiplying occasions of contact between the hospital and persons outside. The aim should be to reduce such occasions to the fewest.

The requirement of an efficient fence is especially needed at

[1] See evidence of Dr Tripe before Royal Commission on Small-Pox and Fever Hospitals, 1882.

a small-pox hospital, owing to the high personal infectivity
of the disease, and to the circumstance that the patients are often
persons of wandering habits, difficult to control. More than one
outbreak of small-pox has originated in the escape of a delirious
patient from a hospital.

The buildings will comprise an administration block in which
the resident caretakers may reside at times when there are
no patients; one or more ward-blocks and the necessary out-
buildings. The number of beds to be provided will depend on
local circumstances; one per 3000 population was suggested as a
standard by Sir G. Buchanan in 1875, but the needs of districts
will vary according to the character of the population, and the
opportunities for introduction of infection. A small permanent
nucleus will suffice for the isolation of the stray cases which occur
from time to time, if there are the means for rapid extension
on an emergency. There is need for small isolation wards at a
small-pox hospital in view of the frequent occurrence of mild
and doubtful cases, which should be isolated promptly, lest they
should be small-pox, but which, unless it is certain that they are
small-pox, should not be exposed to the risk of contracting the
disease from other patients in a large ward. Hence, if only one
ward-block is at first provided it may conveniently take the form
of the late Local Government Board's plan B (8 beds) or plan D
(4 beds). In larger districts where a greater amount of permanent provision is likely to be needed, a block on plan C may
be added for 8 or 12 beds. But the larger the amount of
accommodation provided, and the greater the cost of the hospital,
the less likely is it to be reserved for small-pox emergencies, as
there will be the greater temptation to put a large and costly
hospital to other uses, rather than let it stand empty.

The temporary extensions which may be made on an
emergency may take the form, for summer use, of tents, or of
either of the kinds of temporary buildings mentioned in the
last chapter[1]. It is desirable that platforms of concrete or

[1] The putting up of temporary buildings in proximity to a small-pox hospital full
of acute cases involves considerable danger to the workpeople, and none should be
employed who are not efficiently protected by re-vaccination. An extensive spread of
small-pox took place in 1901 through the agency of men employed in putting up

asphalte should be laid down beforehand, upon which the temporary buildings or tents can be erected when the time comes. The platforms should be of the size and shape for the structures to be erected on them. It will be well that the administration block and out-buildings should be on a scale sufficient to serve for the temporary extensions as well as for the permanent nucleus.

The design and details of the buildings of a small-pox hospital will not differ from those of a hospital for other infectious diseases. Ample cubic space and good ventilation are very necessary.

With a view to prevent the spread of aerial infection the small-pox wards at certain hospitals were formerly so contrived that all the air issuing from the wards should pass through a gas furnace in order that any infective particles which it might contain should be burnt and destroyed[1]. The late Dr F. W. Barry, however, found that abundant living bacteria were still present in the air which had passed through these furnaces, and their use has now been given up, at any rate at the Kendray Hospital Barnsley, which was the best example seen by Dr Barry.

The windows of small-pox wards have, in some cases, been fitted with ruby glass, with a view to carrying out Finsen's red light treatment, but the same object can be obtained at less cost by pasting ruby paper, such as is used by photographers, over the window panes[2].

A steam disinfector is very necessary at a small-pox hospital owing to the persistence with which the infection attaches itself to articles of clothing and bedding.

temporary buildings for the Metropolitan Asylums Board and at certain hospitals in Essex. Tents may for this reason be preferable, when weather permits, to buildings which require more time and labour to erect.

[1] See memorandum by Dr (Sir J.) Burdon Sanderson appended to report of Royal Commission on Small-Pox and Fever Hospitals, 1882.

[2] Dr H. Peck, M.O.H., Chesterfield, says, "My experience of the treatment by red light has made me believe that under it the mortality is lessened; the suffering mitigated; and the permanent disfigurement diminished or avoided, while the average length of the period of detention in hospital is much reduced." Experience at the Metropolitan Asylums Board's hospitals however appears to have been less favourable. Patients subjected to this method of treatment have complained much of depression caused by it.

Aerial convection of Small-pox. By this term is meant the assumption that particulate infectious matter from a hospital containing acute cases of small-pox is on occasion conveyed through the atmosphere in such a way as to infect susceptible people at a considerable distance from the hospital. This view has been the subject of much debate; not that it is disputed that small-pox does often spread among the residents in the neighbourhood of a small-pox hospital, but that the opponents contend that its spread may be sufficiently explained by direct or mediate infection through personal intercourse and leakages of various kinds—likely to be most numerous when the hospital is full—without the need to invoke aerial convection.

The question first arose in connection with small-pox hospitals in London. The Metropolitan Asylums Board first began to isolate small-pox during the great epidemic of 1871, and from that time to 1886 the hospitals used for the purpose were within or on the outskirts of London, surrounded by, or at the edge of, thickly populated areas. In the latter part of 1880 complaints were received by the Local Government Board that an exceptional number of cases of small-pox were occurring around certain hospitals of the Metropolitan Asylums Board, and Mr Power (later Sir W. H. Power, F.R.S.) was instructed to enquire into the circumstances as regards the Fulham Hospital, in the neighbourhood of which a sudden outburst of small-pox occurred in January, 1881. After a long and careful inquiry, Mr Power arrived at the following results, which were entirely unexpected by him at the outset.

" There has been, during each epidemic period, an excessive incidence of small-pox on houses in the neighbourhood of the Fulham Hospital as compared with more distant houses in Chelsea, Fulham and Kensington.

" The percentage of houses invaded in the neighbourhood of the hospital has become gradually smaller as the distance of the houses from the hospital has increased. This gradation has been very exact and very constant.

" Houses upon the chief lines of human intercourse with the hospital have not suffered more than houses lying in other directions from the hospital.

" In point of time there has been a very marked relation
between the varying use of the hospital and the manifestations
of excessive small-pox in the neighbourhood.   This relation
has not shown itself while the use of the hospital has been for
convalescents only.

" The appearance of excessive small-pox in houses around
the hospital has never been delayed until the hospital has
become full or nearly full.   It has been always most remarkable when admissions to the hospital were beginning to increase
rapidly.

" On comparison of different epidemics an almost constant
ratio is observed between the amount of the hospital operations
and the degree of excess of small-pox on the neighbourhood.

" The machinery of the hospital administration, with inclusion
of defects in that machinery, does not account for the peculiarity
of small-pox incidence within the three parishes of Chelsea,
Fulham and Kensington since the establishment of the hospital.

" There must have been some condition or conditions operating
to produce the observed distribution of small-pox around the
hospital that have pertained to the hospital as such, and that
have been in excess of the conditions for small-pox extension as
usually recognised."

From these results ascertained by him Mr Power was led to
make the suggestion that the excessive incidence of small-pox
on the area surrounding the Fulham Hospital, and especially the
sudden outburst in January 1881, could be best explained by the
hypothesis of a dissemination of particulate infection through the
atmosphere (for which the meteorological conditions in January
1881 were especially favourable), coupled with a higher potency
of the infection resulting from the bringing together of many
cases in the acute stage of the disease.

The sequel was the appointment in November 1881 of a
Royal Commission to inquire respecting Small-Pox and Fever
Hospitals, who reported in 1882.   Their report states that evidence of the spread of small-pox around the hospital had been
received with respect not only to the Fulham Hospital but also
to those at Hampstead, Homerton, Stockwell and Deptford;
and that injunctions had been issued by the Courts forbidding

the use of the Hampstead Hospital for small-pox cases, and limiting that of the Fulham Hospital to cases of small-pox residing within a mile of the hospital. They say:

"That by some means or other the Asylums' Hospitals in their present shape cause an increase of small-pox in their neighbourhoods appears to us clearly established by the experience of these five hospitals during the past ten years."

Against a belief in widely extending atmospheric dissemination they mentioned, however,

"That the number of facts supporting it is at present too small;

"That the chief of these facts have been observed in the case of only one hospital;

"That the evidence in disproof of sufficient personal communication in the neighbourhood of this hospital is necessarily very negative and incomplete;

"That the immunity of persons living near small-pox hospitals, if guarded from all, even indirect, personal communication with their inmates, is quite inconsistent with the belief in infection by particles carried far through the air."

They quoted several instances of large institutions situated within short distances (90 ft. to ¼ mile) from small-pox hospitals, among the inmates of which there had nevertheless been very little small-pox.

They recommended that for the mild and convalescent cases of small-pox two or three hospitals in the country should be provided, and for those who were too ill to bear a long journey that small hospitals of 30 or 40 beds with separate administrative blocks should be maintained within the precincts of the fever hospitals, but they say

"It is evidently of paramount importance that the areas of the small-pox wards, as well as their administration, should be rigorously separated from those of the fever hospitals."

A later report on the influence of the Fulham Small-Pox Hospital on the neighbourhood surrounding it was made by Mr Power in 1885. Fulham Hospital had been closed for small-pox cases from December 1881 to May 1884, and during that time there had been very little small-pox in Chelsea, Fulham

and Kensington, and certainly no excess of incidence on the
neighbourhood of the hospital. The managers had remodelled
their administration with the view of reducing and more strictly
supervising the communications between the hospital and the
outside world, and an efficient ambulance service had been
organised by the Metropolitan Asylums Board. The hospital
was reopened for small-pox on May 15th, 1884, and in the fort-
night ending 7th June there was a great increase of small-pox in
Chelsea, Fulham and Kensington ; the number of houses invaded,
which in the two preceding fortnights had been 12 and 9,
suddenly rose to 37, of which 25 were within a radius of one
mile from the hospital. From that time to Sept. 13 there were
received into hospital 162 small-pox patients, but the number

*Table showing the percentages of houses invaded with small-pox
in two periods of 1884 within distances from Fulham Hospital.*

Periods, 1884	Percentages of houses invaded with small-pox within distances from Fulham Hospital					
	Under ¼ mile	¼—½ mile	½—¾ mile	¾—1 mile	Under 1 mile	1—3½ miles. Rest of three parishes
Non-hospital, Jan. 1—May 25	—	·02	·07	·02	·05	·06
Hospital, May 25—Sept. 13	·70	·76	·40	·25	·45	·21

under treatment at one time exceeded 35 on three occasions only.
Nevertheless there was during this period, as in 1881, a graduated
excess of small-pox on the neighbourhood of the hospital, and
this excess began to be evident when the total admissions to the
hospital had not exceeded nine.

After 1885 no more small-pox cases were treated in the
hospitals of the Metropolitan Asylums Board in London, all
being taken down the river to hospital ships and hospitals
near Dartford. The Small-Pox Hospital was not removed from
Highgate until 1896, but its operations were on a small scale.

The sequel has been very striking. Before the removal of
the small-pox hospitals out of London small-pox was constantly

present, becoming epidemic about every fifth year. After 1885 there was a sudden change; the small-pox death-rate, which was 332 per million inhabitants in 1885, fell to 5 per million in 1886 (including deaths of Londoners in small-pox hospitals outside the Metropolis), and, except for minor epidemics in 1893—5 and 1901—2, has continued below 10 per million ever since; the mortality from small-pox in several recent years having indeed been nil. See diagram on next page.

It need not, however, be supposed that the practical extinction of small-pox as an endemic disease in London has been brought about solely by extra-mural isolation; other improvements in sanitary administration, and probably a milder type of the disease, have no doubt had a share in the result.

But this advantage to London has not been gained without some detriment to the locality to which the London small-pox cases are removed. In a paper read before the Epidemiological Society on April 18th, 1902, Dr Thresh says: "Prior to the floating hospitals being established near Purfleet, small-pox was little more prevalent in the Orsett district than in the remainder of the county (of Essex), and only from one-third to one-fourth as prevalent as in the Metropolis. The change since then has been most marked, for on the same basis the disease has been seven times more prevalent in Orsett than in the remainder of the county, and 2½ times more prevalent than in London."

The greater prevalence of small-pox in the Orsett district began in 1884, the year in which small-pox cases were first brought to the hospital ships, and continued in the following year; it was also observed in the years 1893—5, during which there was a minor epidemic of small-pox in London and many cases were brought to the ships; and on a still greater scale in 1901—2, when there was a larger epidemic in London. The place most affected has been Purfleet, a village in the parish of West Thurrock immediately opposite the hospital ships, and to the E.N.E. of them, i.e. in the path of the prevalent winds from the ships. The ships are moored near to the Kentish shore, the adjacent land being uninhabited marshes, and are separated from Purfleet by nearly the whole breadth of the Thames estuary, here half a mile wide. In the years 1893—5 there was a certain

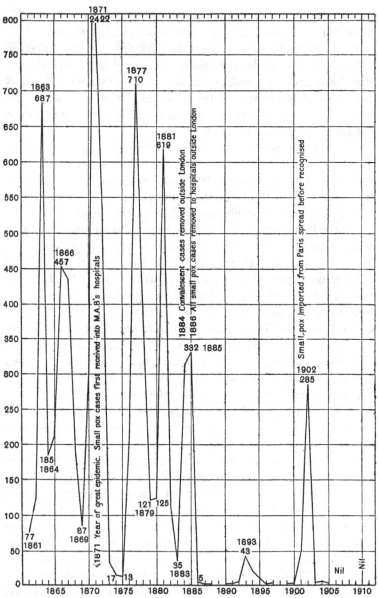

Diagram showing for London the death rates from small-pox per million of the
population from 1861 to 1911. (Deaths of London inhabitants in small-pox
hospitals outside London included.)

amount of intercommunication between the ships and the Essex shore, but before 1901 this intercommunication had been entirely cut off. Between Nov. 1901 and June 1902 the average daily number of patients on the ships was 164, the minimum and maximum numbers being 97 and 271. Severe cases preponderated, the milder cases being transferred to the Gore Farm Hospital in Kent within a few days of their arrival. During the epidemic period several instances occurred in which members of the crew of ships which had moored for a while in the river near the hospital ships were taken ill of small-pox about 12 days later, but the lads and staff of the training ship Cornwall, moored in the river within $\frac{1}{2}$ mile N. of the hospital ships, practically escaped, being protected by vaccination and re-vaccination.

At a number of other places a special prevalence of small-pox has been observed in the neighbourhood of hospitals in which many cases were collected, and has been attributed by investigators to spread of the disease through the atmosphere. On the other hand this view has been by no means generally accepted by medical officers of health, and discussions have taken place from time to time at which arguments against the aerial convection of small-pox have been ably put forward.

The considerations adduced in favour of aerial convection of small-pox may be thus summed up:

An excessive incidence of small-pox has in numerous instances been found to occur around hospitals in which many acute cases of the disease are collected together.

This incidence is graduated according to distance from the hospital; a greater percentage of the houses within $\frac{1}{4}$ mile from the hospital being invaded than of those between $\frac{1}{4}$ and $\frac{1}{2}$ mile, and a greater percentage of the latter than of those in more distant zones.

The prevalence of small-pox in the neighbourhood of the hospital bears a relation to the extent of the operations of the hospital; it is greatest when the number of acute cases under treatment is rapidly increasing.

The disuse for small-pox of one hospital with the substituted use of another has led, as at London, to a transference of small-pox prevalence from the neighbourhood of the former to that of the latter.

The excessive incidence of small-pox in the neighbourhood of the hospital is not sufficiently explained by personal communications incidental to the working of the hospital, or by leakages owing to defects in the working, and has persisted when such communications have been reduced to a minimum and surrounded with every safeguard against the carriage of infection.

The ordinary communications without special precautions have little effect in spreading small-pox from a hospital in which the cases are few or only in the convalescent stage.

In many of the cases occurring in the special zone the most careful inquiry fails to discover any personal communication, direct or indirect, with the hospital.

That communication, direct or indirect, with the hospital can be ascertained to have taken place in a few cases, does not disprove that the infection may have been air-borne in others. It is not contended that persons exposed to aerial infection are immune to infection conveyed by other channels; the hypothesis only professes to account for the excess of incidence, not for the whole incidence within the special area.

The houses nearest to the hospital would not necessarily be those most liable to be affected by personal communications. At Glasgow the earlier cases in the hospital came from a distant quarter of the city, and visitors to the hospital would come from that quarter rather than from the one nearest the hospital which only became infected later on. At Gateshead the spread of small-pox took place in another district having little or no communication with the Gateshead hospital. At Purfleet the locality which suffered was separated from the hospital ships by a tidal river half a mile wide.

Instances in which small-pox has not spread from a hospital do not necessarily disprove that it has done so in other cases. It is not contended that such spread takes place in all cases, but only under certain conditions, especially when many acute cases are collected together. Few, if any, instances are recorded in which many acute cases of small-pox have been under treatment

at one time in a hospital situated in a populous neighbourhood, without more or less prevalence of small-pox occurring
around it.

Escape of institutions within the special area has in some
instances been accounted for by the inmates being protected by
vaccination.

All states of the weather are not equally favourable to
atmospheric convection. Rain and strong winds would wash
down or disperse infective particles. The most favourable
meteorological conditions are calm, cool, misty weather, with
a gentle and steady movement of the air. Observation shows
that in such weather particulate matter, *e.g.* smoke from a factory
chimney, may be carried through the air for distances of a mile
or more with comparatively little dispersion.

Particles such as volcanic dust, spores and pollen grains[1] can
be conveyed suspended in the atmosphere for great distances.
Bacteria experimentally sprayed into the air have been recovered
at distances up to 600 metres.

In some instances, as at Purfleet and Gateshead, the spread
of small-pox has distinctly followed the direction of the prevalent
wind.

Arguments used against the hypothesis of aerial convection
are:

A more obvious explanation of the prevalence of small-pox
around a small-pox hospital can be found in direct or mediate
infection conveyed by personal communications, such as ambulance journeys, visits of friends to patients, visits paid by
nurses when off duty, calls of tradesmen and workmen, staff
residing off the premises, and leakages of various kinds, as well
as by "contacts" and "missed cases."

Communications of these kinds would be more numerous
with houses situated near the hospital than with those farther

[1] In some plants cross-fertilisation is effected by pollen grains wafted by the wind;
in other plants pollen grains are carried from flower to flower by insects. Impreg-
nation by air-borne pollen may take place over a considerable distance as in the case
of diœcious trees, such as poplars and willows; but a much larger amount of pollen
has to be produced where the pollen is wind-borne than suffices when it is conveyed
more directly by insects.

off, and thus the incidence of small-pox would be graduated according to distance from the hospital.

Such communications would be more frequent in proportion as the number of patients in the hospital became larger, and at times when it was very full the administration would be strained, and regulations intended to prevent the spread of infection would be apt to be disregarded. It is at such times that the spread of small-pox around hospitals has occurred.

A necessary condition, it has been said, for scientific proof of atmospheric dissemination of contagion through a circle of a mile radius would be the elimination of all means of ordinary communication in the intervening space. If one case of small-pox within the special area around the hospital can be accounted for by infection through personal communication, the inference is that other cases in the same area can be similarly accounted for by communications which have taken place but are not discoverable by later inquiry.

Difficulty in tracing such communications arises from the inquiry being made some time after the event, and when circumstances apparently trivial, but which may have been important, have been forgotten. Also the nurses and employees of the hospital would not be likely to "give themselves away" by owning to carelessness and breaches of the regulations.

Instances have occurred in which there has been no special incidence of small-pox around a small-pox hospital. Institutions in its neighbourhood but having no communication with it have escaped wholly or with a few cases only. Patients in the fever wards at the same hospital have in some instances escaped.

The apparent special incidence of small-pox cases in the neighbourhood of small-pox hospitals, shown by spot maps, may be merely a matter of coincidence or of density of population. At Liverpool there was such an apparent special incidence around a hospital which was not used for small-pox at all.

"Hospital influence" is only manifested at times when the hospital contains many cases of small-pox, and this is, from the nature of the case, a time when the disease has an epidemic tendency to spread apart from such influence.

Infection from a small-pox hospital reaching a person at a distance through the air would be so diluted that the dose would be insufficient to overcome the natural powers of resistance of the body.

The modern growth of knowledge has tended to discredit the idea of aerial infection. Diseases such as influenza and diphtheria, which were formerly supposed to be capable of being conveyed long distances through the air, are now known to be propagated from person to person. In antiseptic surgery the precautions at first adopted against infection reaching wounds through the air have been found unnecessary.

Rules founded on the hypothesis of aerial convection are in practice vexatious and unnecessary.

The question of the aerial convection of small-pox is not one capable of strict proof or disproof; the arguments on either side being subject to the proverbial difficulty of proving a negative; we can only select the hypothesis which seems best to fit with the facts. But if we reject the possibility of aerial dissemination, and maintain that the spread of the disease around hospitals can in all cases be explained by direct or mediate infection through personal channels, we must be prepared to admit that such channels may be so elusive and difficult of control that able investigators and administrators have often been unable to discover them, or to frame and enforce regulations sufficient to arrest them. Or, as an alternative, we may suppose that the propagation takes place by some other means not at present known.

But the acceptance or rejection of the hypothesis of aerial convection of small-pox does not in practice make so much difference as might be supposed. In the words of Dr M°Vail: "The practical conclusion of this whole question may be said to have already been arrived at. Small-pox hospitals are not now erected in the midst of towns, and those already in existence are being more and more sparingly used. Indeed, where the power of aerial convection is still doubted, it seems to be assumed that the prevention of personal communication is impracticable, and that accidents incident to the system of

hospital treatment of small-pox within populous districts must
be accepted as inevitable, so that the only remedy under the one
theory as under the other, is the removal of such institutions to
a distance from populous places."

To this conclusion Dr Thresh adds that it may be necessary
to avoid having large institutions with consequent large concentration of patients, and therefore of infective material, by
substituting for them a number of smaller hospitals or a number
of tent encampments in which this concentration of infection
cannot occur.   For isolation on a large scale he recommends the
provision of permanent administrative buildings and the scattering of the patients over a large area in properly constructed and
equipped marquees, none containing more than 40 patients.
The erection of these during an epidemic would involve the
employment of the minimum number of men and the expenditure of the minimum amount of money.

BIBLIOGRAPHY

Bristowe and Holmes.   The hospitals of the United Kingdom, in report of
    Medical Officer to Privy Council. 1863.
Buchanan, Sir G.   English hospitals in their sanitary aspects. 1875.
Report of Hospitals Commission. 1882.
Thorne.   Hospital Report. 1882.   Containing Mr, now Sir William Power's
    original report on the influence of the Fulham Small-Pox Hospital on
    the neighbourhood.
Davies, D. S.   Diphtheria and Small-pox, an epidemiological contrast.
    Public Health, March, 1907.
Parsons.   Hospital Report. 1912.
—— Report on Small-pox at Ivybridge : and spread of infection from rags
    at Paper Mills.   Report of M.O. Local Government Board. 1886.
—— Memorandum on Epidemics of Small-pox among Colonies of Navvies.
    Report of M.O. Local Government Board. 1905—6.
Armstrong, H. E.   Reports on Small-pox and Vagrants. 1903—4.
Barry, F. W.   Report to the Local Government Board on means for de-
    stroying infection in the air issuing from Small-pox hospitals. 1894.
Peck, H.   Small-pox treatment by red light. Public Health, April, 1904,
    and Feb. 1907.
Power, Sir W. H.   Fulham Hospital Report and reports in annual volumes
    of Medical Officer, Local Government Board, for 1884 and 1885.
Annual Report of the Medical Officer of the Local Government Board for

1886, containing reports by Mr Power, on Statistics of Small-pox incidence upon the Registration districts of London relatively to the operations of Small-pox hospitals in the Metropolis, and on the behaviour of Small-pox at West Ham in the epidemic of 1884—5.

Transactions of Society of Medical Officers of Health. Jan. 16, 1885. "Are Small-pox hospitals necessarily (*per se*) a source of danger to the surrounding population?" Papers by Drs E. T. Wilson, Gwynn and Tripe.

Murphy, Sir S. Annual Report of M.O.H. for St Pancras. 1884.

Notes on an outbreak of Small-pox at Nottingham in 1887—8, by Dr B. A. Whitelegge. Practitioner, Vol. XLI. No 1. (Small-pox at Nottingham is also dealt with by Dr E. C. Seaton in an article on "The Influence of Small-pox hospitals," in the Transactions of the Epidemiol. Society, N.S. Vol. II. 1883, in a sense contrary to aerial convection.)

Reports of Registrar General.

The Metropolitan Asylums Board of London and its work. 1900.

Thresh, J. C. Small-pox hospitals and the spread of infection. Trans. Epidemiological Society, Vol. XXI. 1902.

Niven, J. Annual Report on health of Oldham. 1892.

Gornall, G. Report on the epidemic of Small-pox in 1892—3 in the borough of Warrington.

Savill. Report on the outbreak of Small-pox in the borough of Warrington in 1892—3. (Appendix V to Final Report of the Royal Commission on Vaccination.)

McVail, J. C. The aerial convection of Small-pox from Hospitals. Transactions of Epidemiological Society, N.S. Vol. XIII. 1893.

(In this paper Dr McVail mentions a controversy on the subject between Dr Haygarth of Chester and Dr Waterhouse of Cambridge, Massachusetts, at the end of the 18th century, and also a paper by Sir John Rose Cormack in the Edinburgh Medical Review of 1881, showing that facts relating to the spread of small-pox around hospitals had been observed in Paris.)

Low, R. Bruce. Report on the prevalence of Small-pox in and around the borough of Hastings, in annual volume of the Medical Officer, Local Government Board. 1894—5.

Evans, Arnold. The aerial convection of Small-pox. British Medical Journal, Aug. 18, 1894.

Chalmers. Reports on Small-pox in Glasgow. 1900—2 and 1903—4.

Buchanan, G. S. Report on epidemic Small-pox in the Union of Orsett. Annual Report of Medical Officer of Local Government Board. 1903. Also a paper in Transactions of Epidemiological Society. 1905.

Annual Report of the Medical Officer of the Local Government Board for 1904—5 containing reports by Dr Buchanan on Small-pox in Gateshead and Felling in relation to Sheriff Hill Hospital and by Dr R. J. Reece on Small-pox and Small-pox Hospitals at Liverpool.

Journal of Royal Sanitary Institute.   Vols. XXV and XXVI.

Rundle.   Transactions of Epidemiological Section, Royal Society of
    Medicine, May, 1912.

Chapin, C. V.   The importance of contact infection.   American Journal of
    Public Hygiene, Aug. 1910.

Campbell, J.   The Gloucester Small-pox epidemic.   Public Health, April,
    1897.

Coupland, S.   Report on outbreak of Small-pox at Gloucester.   Appendix
    VII to Final report of Royal Commission on Vaccination.   1897.

Collie, A.   Small-pox and its diffusion.   1912.

CHAPTER X

PORT SANITARY HOSPITALS

PORT Sanitary Authorities are constituted of representatives
of the several riparian districts adjoining the port, and they
have in regard to ships similar sanitary powers to those which
Town and District Councils exercise on shore, including the
power to provide hospitals.   They have special duties under the
Regulations of the Ministry of Health with respect to the
treatment of persons affected with cholera, yellow fever and
plague, and for preventing the spread of such diseases, and
are required to make provision for the reception of persons
suffering from these maladies.   They may also have to deal
with any of the ordinary infectious diseases occurring on
board ship, and particularly with small-pox, which is frequently imported by vessels, especially from Russia, Southern
Europe and Mediterranean countries and South America;
also with malarial fevers, and parasitic maladies, which are not
likely to spread under present circumstances in this country,
as well as the more ordinary diseases.   These diseases may
occur on board ship among the crew, many of whom are
foreigners, often Orientals; or among the passengers, who at
certain ports include many emigrants from Eastern Europe,
often uncleanly in person and coming from places where epidemics are frequent.

The system of quarantine—that is detaining an infected or

suspected vessel, with all on board, for a period sufficiently long to cover the period of incubation, after the termination of the last case or after leaving an infected port—has long fallen into desuetude in this country and was finally abolished by the Public Health Act, 1896. The present procedure is that a ship reported by the customs officer to be infected with plague cholera or yellow fever, or suspected to be infected or to have come from an infected place, is boarded by the port medical officer of health who, if he finds the ship to be infected, gives a certificate to that effect, and the ship is then required to be moored at an appointed place, and no person on board is allowed to leave the ship until he has been examined by the medical officer of health. Every person certified by the medical officer to be suffering from plague, cholera or yellow fever is to be removed, if his condition permits, to hospital or some other suitable place appointed for the purpose, and must remain there until certified to be free from the disease. Persons suffering from any illness which the medical officer of health suspects may prove to be plague, cholera or yellow fever may either be detained on board for a period not exceeding two days, or may be taken to hospital and detained there for a like period. Other persons on board such a ship are permitted to land if they satisfy the medical officer of health as to their names, places of destination and intended addresses at such places, and notice of their coming is to be sent to the local authority in whose district their place of destination is situated. If a ship, though not infected, has passengers on board who are in a filthy or otherwise unwholesome condition, or has come from a place infected with cholera, yellow fever or plague, persons on board such ship may, on a certificate by the medical officer of health, be forbidden to land until they have satisfied him as to their names, places of destination and addresses. After disinfection, and any necessary measures for the destruction of rats and for dealing with bilge water, water ballast and drinking water have been carried out, the ship is allowed to go free.

As regards infectious diseases other than cholera, yellow fever and plague the legal powers of local authorities (port and other) for the removal to hospital and the detention there of persons suffering from infectious disease, who are on board any ship or vessel, are referred to in Chapter XI. The powers of local authorities relating to infectious diseases and hospitals under §§ 120, 121, 124, 125, 128, 131, 132 and 133 of the Public Health Act, 1875, are extended to ships by the Public Health (Ships) Act, 1885.

The owner or master of a ship is liable for the medical treatment of a seaman taken ill in the service of the ship.

Floating Hospitals. The choice between a floating hospital and one on shore will depend on local circumstances, and more especially on the relative feasibility of obtaining a convenient and suitable mooring-place or site on shore, but a hospital on shore is generally to be preferred as being more easily administered, and accessible night and day and in all weathers and states of the tide, unless indeed it is on an island, as it has sometimes been placed for the sake of better isolation. The requirements for a port hospital on shore will not differ materially from the usual requirements of an isolation hospital, but it will be convenient for it to be placed near the shore, with a landing place for cases brought by water[1].

The arrangements made for the reception of cholera cases on occasions of threatened invasions of that disease have often been very crude; examples were given in Chapter III. The chief objects held in view seem to have been that it should be near the shipping centres, that it could be provided in a short time and at small cost.

Examples of port sanitary hospitals which are on shore are those of the London, Liverpool, Weymouth and Hartlepool Port Sanitary Authorities. Cardiff has a cholera hospital on the Flat Holm island in the Bristol Channel.

In choosing the mooring-place for a floating hospital the points to be sought are a safe anchorage, convenient of approach but well out of the navigation channel, and not near a populous locality on shore. If sufficiently near the shore water and gas

---

[1] In two instances the hospital of a port sanitary authority has been used also as the isolation hospital for the general use of the constituent districts, but this arrangement has not been found to work well. In many cases the hospital of a riparian district is used by arrangement for port cases.

may be laid on in pipes, otherwise the supply of water will have to be conveyed in a tank or barrels by boat.

A floating hospital may be either a structure specially designed as a hospital or an existing vessel adapted by alterations for the purpose. Hospitals of the first kind consist of wooden ward-blocks erected on a platform or deck which rests on floating pontoons, with administrative buildings on the same platform or on another vessel moored near it and connected by a gangway. Examples of this form of floating hospital are those of the river Tyne and the river Tees Port Sanitary Authorities, and also the Castalia hospital ship of the Metropolitan Asylums Board, in which the understructure was a twin-keeled vessel originally constructed for the cross-channel traffic; see Chapter XVI.

At other ports vessels of various sorts and sizes from a barge or lighter up to a steamship of 2000 tons burden have been used as hospital ships, as at Plymouth, Southampton, Portsmouth (formerly), Ipswich and Harwich. Wooden cabins for wards may be erected on the upper deck and rooms below may be used for administrative purposes. Floating hospitals, however, are not now so popular as they were at one time.

In a report to the West Ham Town Council in 1894 Dr Sanders gives figures of the respective cost of a hospital ship as compared with a hospital on land, from which it appears that the former is likely to be the most expensive, both in first cost and in cost of maintenance.

BIBLIOGRAPHY

Thorne. Hospital Report. 1882.

Hospital Return. 1895.

Regulations of the Local Government Board, *re* Cholera, Yellow Fever and Plague. 9th September, 1907.

Annual Report of the Medical Officer of the Local Government Board, 1908—9, containing report by Dr Theodore Thomson on the Board's Sanitary Survey of the coast line of England and Wales, 1907—8.

Sanders, C. The relative cost of land and ship small-pox hospitals. Public Health, Jan. 1895.

Southampton Port Sanatorium. Public Health, Nov. 1894.

CHAPTER XI

REMOVAL OF PATIENTS TO HOSPITAL

Legal powers of removal. The Sanitary Act, 1866, which gave to "Sewer Authorities" power to provide within their district hospitals or temporary places for the reception of the sick (see p. 14) gave to "Nuisance Authorities," by § 26 *a*, power of removal to such places. Thus the functions of provision of a hospital, and of the removal of patients to it, were placed in the hands of different authorities; an order could only be made for removal to a hospital actually within the district of the Nuisance Authority, and no penalty was fixed for non-compliance.

These defects were amended by § 124, Public Health Act, 1875, which applies in England and Wales outside London.

> Where any suitable hospital or place for the reception of the sick is provided within the district of a local authority, or within a convenient distance of such district, any person who is suffering from any dangerous infectious disorder, and is without proper lodging or accommodation, or lodged in a room occupied by more than one family, or is on board any ship or vessel, may, on a certificate signed by a legally qualified medical practitioner, and with the consent of the superintending body of such hospital or place, be removed, by order of any justice, to such hospital or place at the cost of the local authority; and any person so suffering, who is lodged in any common lodging-house, may, with the like consent and on a like certificate, be so removed by order of the local authority.
>
> An order under this section may be addressed to such constable or officer of the local authority as the justice or local authority making the same may think expedient; and any person who wilfully disobeys or obstructs the execution of such order shall be liable to a penalty not exceeding ten pounds.

It was also provided by § 125:

> Any local authority may make regulations (to be approved of by the Local Government Board) for removing to any hospital to which such authority are entitled to remove patients, and for keeping in such hospital so long as may be necessary, any persons brought within their district by any ship or boat who are infected with a dangerous infectious disorder, and such regulations may impose on offenders against the same reasonable penalties not exceeding forty shillings for each offence.

The Act does not provide for the detention of infected

persons in hospital in other cases, but such detention can usually be secured indirectly by pointing out that a penalty is incurred, under § 126, by any person who while suffering from any dangerous infectious disorder wilfully exposes himself without proper precautions against spreading the said disorder in any street, public place, shop, inn, or public conveyance.

§ 22, Poor Law Amendment Act, 1867, gives power to the Guardians, or, when they are not sitting, to the master of a workhouse to detain in the workhouse any poor person suffering from bodily disease of an infectious or contagious character, whom the medical officer of the workhouse may report in writing to be not in a proper state to leave the workhouse without danger to himself or others. This section is not limited to notifiable diseases, and would apparently authorise the detention of *e.g.* a case of advanced phthisis, or of venereal disease or itch.

A doubt formerly existed whether the words in § 124, Public Health Act, 1875, "without proper lodging or accommodation," referred merely to the lack of such accommodation as was needed for the patient's own welfare, or whether they might be held to include cases where the patient had accommodation of a sort, but not such as to enable him to be properly isolated.

In the case, however, of Warwick *v.* Graham (80 L.T. 773), it was held by the Queen's Bench Division of the High Court, that the words in question refer to the protection of other persons from infection, and not merely to the welfare of the patient himself.

§ 65 of the Public Health Acts Amendment Act, 1907 (where it is in force), makes the point clear by declaring that § 124, Public Health Act, 1875, shall extend and apply to all cases of persons suffering from any dangerous infectious disease, and being in or upon any house or premises where such persons cannot be effectually isolated so as to prevent the spread of the disease. (The expression "infectious disease" in this section is however limited by § 13 to those diseases to which the Infectious Diseases (Notification) Act, 1889, for the time being applies within the district.)

In London powers of removal are given by § 66, Public Health (London) Act, 1891 as follows:

(1) A person suffering from any dangerous infectious

P.   10 disease[1] who is without proper lodging or accommodation, or is lodged in any tent or van or is on board any vessel may, on a certificate signed by a legally qualified medical practitioner and with the consent of the superintending body of the hospital to which he is to be removed, be removed by order of a justice and at the cost of the sanitary authority of the district where such person is found, to any hospital in or within a convenient distance of London ; (2) provides for the carrying out of the order, and (3) gives power to make byelaws for keeping in the hospital persons brought into the district by any vessel.

By § 67 (1), a justice on being satisfied that a person suffering from any dangerous infectious disease is in a hospital, and would not on leaving the hospital be provided with lodging or accommodation in which proper precautions could be taken to prevent the spreading of the disease by such person, may direct such person to be maintained in the hospital at the cost of the Metropolitan Asylums Managers, during the time limited by the justice. Any justice may enlarge the time as often as appears to him necessary for preventing the spread of the disease.

It will be observed that the cases in which compulsory removal to hospital is explicitly sanctioned by the law are comparatively few, and this want of power of compulsory removal is sometimes adduced by unwilling local authorities as a reason for not providing an isolation hospital. But it is found in practice that resort to compulsory powers is rarely necessary. Where a comfortable and attractive hospital has been provided, and is under management which commands public confidence, and where its use is not impeded by heavy charges, people find out its advantages through their own experience or that of their neighbours, and any prejudices which may at first be entertained against it tend to disappear. In places where such prejudice has been expected to be met

This expression, by § 38, is limited to the diseases compulsorily notifiable under § 55 (8), viz. small-pox, cholera, diphtheria, membranous croup, erysipelas, the disease known as scarlatina or scarlet fever, and the fevers known as typhus, typhoid, enteric, relapsing, continued, or puerperal ; but may be applied to any other infectious disease by order.

with it has sometimes been found useful, when the hospital has been completed, to inaugurate it by a public ceremony, and to allow it to remain open for public inspection for a few days before any patients are admitted. On the other hand it has sometimes come about that a hospital has incurred unmerited discredit through the first cases admitted into it happening to prove fatal; it might therefore be prudent to refrain at first from removing to it, unless under circumstances of urgency, patients whose condition was such as to threaten the occurrence of such a mischance.

But with modern improvements in means of communication and transport, and with increased experience of the advantages of hospital treatment, as regards not only the welfare of the patient, but also the avoidance of the inconveniences and dis- abilities entailed by the presence of infection in the household, the objection to removal of patients from their homes has much diminished. Indeed popular feeling has gone so far in the opposite direction that it is now sometimes complained of as a hardship by parents if their children, when suffering from an infectious disease, have to be treated at home; and the cost of their maintenance in such circumstances has even been claimed, though probably it could not be recovered.

§ 131, Public Health Act, 1875, being in terms permissive and not compulsory there would seem to be no obligation upon a sanitary authority to provide hospital accommodation for a case of infectious disease, if they do not possess it. But whether an authority, who have provided a hospital, may refuse to admit any person resident in their district suffering from infectious disease, for whose admission application may be made, is not clear in view of the case of The Queen v. Mayor and Corporation of Rawtenstall (*Times*, 2 Aug. 1894):

"The guardians of the Haslingden Union had provided a hospital separate from but in connection with the workhouse premises, for cases of infectious disease, but they were of opinion that there was risk in admitting infectious cases to such hospital, and they applied to the defendants to receive into their hospital (provided under the Public Health Act, 1875, § 131) pauper patients who were inhabitants of the borough. They consented to do so, the guardians agreeing to pay for the maintenance of the patients.

"Subsequently a dispute arose between the guardians and the defendants as to rate of charge, and the defendants refused to take pauper patients into their hospital. *Held* that it was the duty of the Corporation as long as they had the requisite accommodation to receive into the hospital any inhabitants of the borough who are suffering from infectious disease, whether or not they are paupers; but under § 132 of the Public Health Act, 1875, they are empowered to recover the cost of maintenance in the hospital from non-pauper patients when they are able to pay, and in the case of pauper patients from the guardians."

This judgment need not perhaps be held to mean that so long as there is a bed vacant in the hospital, the hospital authority are bound to admit every applicant from the district, irrespective of the need for separating different infectious diseases, or for reserving beds for specially urgent cases, or cases of a different kind. The Local Government Board have said that they have no authority to determine the question, but that they think that the local authority have a discretion under which they may give the preference as regards admission to the cases which are most urgent.

Instances have occurred in which the too consistent application of the principle "First come, first served" has led to the hospital being filled with trivial cases of scarlet fever, to the exclusion of other and more serious diseases, and of cases more urgently needing isolation.

Charge for admission to isolation hospital. The Public Health Act, 1875, contains the following section:

> Any expenses incurred by a local authority in maintaining in a hospital, or in a temporary place for the reception of the sick (whether or not belonging to such authority), a patient who is not a pauper, shall be deemed to be a debt due from such patient to the local authority, and may be recovered from him at any time within six months after his discharge from such hospital or place of reception, or from his estate in the event of his dying in such hospital or place.

It has been usually considered that the above words "may be recovered" allow the local authority an option whether they will or will not make a charge for the use of the hospital, and many local authorities admit cases from their own district under ordinary circumstances free of charge. The above was also the view of the Local Government Board, and in their Memorandum on the provision of Isolation Hospital accommodation, they advise:

> An isolation hospital being intended primarily for the protection of the public at large rather than for the benefit of individuals, it is undesirable that admission should be subject to restrictive charges and conditions which may tend to prevent the use of the hospital by the poorer portion of the community; that is to say, by those who have the least facilities for isolation and treatment at their own homes. In some districts, however, *e.g.* at health resorts, it may be advisable to provide special accommodation of a superior kind, such as private wards, for persons willing to pay for it.

An opinion has however been given by an eminent counsel that, as it is the duty of a local authority to recover all debts due to them, the words "shall be deemed to be a debt due from such patient to the local authority" make it imperative on the latter to take steps in all cases for the recovery of the cost of maintenance. Any doubt on this point may however be removed by the local authority obtaining the powers of § 60, Public Health Acts Amendment Act, 1907, which provides that nothing in § 132, Public Health Act, 1875, shall require the local authority to recover the cost of maintenance from a patient who is not a pauper, where the local authority have satisfied themselves that the circumstances of the case are such as to justify the remission of the debt.

But the powers given by § 132, Public Health Act, 1875, for the recovery of the cost of maintenance in hospital are in practice comparatively limited, as it appears to be only the patient himself or his estate that is made liable for them, and the great majority of patients in an isolation hospital are children, dependents, and persons not in a position to pay. The Courts have decided that in the absence of a contract to pay, express or implied, the section places no statutory liability on a parent in respect of his child, or on the managers of a charitable institution in respect of inmates[1], and probably the

---

[1] In Isle of Thanet Hospital Board *v.* Farquhar, reported in *Public Health*, September, 1904, it was held that the charitable guardians of children who send

same view would hold with respect to employers and their servants. It seems also to be doubtful whether, in the absence of an agreement, guardians of the poor are liable for the maintenance of pauper patients, unless the hospital is one provided under the Isolation Hospitals Act, 1893, in which case § 19 (1) of that Act makes the point clear.

To meet this difficulty local authorities who desired to secure payment for the use of their hospital have sometimes required as a condition of admission that payment of expenses should be guaranteed in writing by some responsible person before removal of the case. But the requirement of such a guarantee has been found to involve delay in removal, and frequent refusal of the hospital for the very cases in which isolation was most needed. In one instance the adoption of a scale of charges, and the requirement of a guarantee of payment, was followed by no admissions into the hospital during a period of 11 years[1]. The general experience appears to be that the collection of the small amounts, which in ordinary cases residents in the district can afford to pay, entails more trouble than the proceeds are worth[2] and that the fact of a charge being made,

---

them to the hospital of a local authority while suffering from an infectious disease are not "patients" within the meaning of § 132 of the Public Health Act, 1875, and cannot be made liable for the expense of maintaining the children, unless there is a contract, express or implied, binding them to pay these expenses.

[1] The scale of charges, which had been adopted, was:

Scale I. for occupiers of houses rated above £10 per annum.

    Children under 5 years of age, 10s. per week.

    Children 5 years of age and under 12, £1 per week.

    Persons 12 years of age and upwards, £2 per week.

Scale II. for occupiers of houses rated at or under £10 per annum, and for domestic servants, indoor apprentices, and shop assistants.

    Children under 5 years of age, 5s. per week.

    Children 5 years of age and under 12, 10s. per week.

    Persons 12 years of age and upwards, £1 per week.

The charges included food, nursing, medical attendance and all other necessaries.

[2] In a report made in 1906, Dr Jordan, medical officer of health to the Heaton Norris Urban District, states that during the years 1901—6, 197 cases of scarlet fever occurred, of which 85 were removed to hospital, and out of these 17 might have been charged for. If a charge for these, varying according to the patients' means from 10s. 6d. to £1. 10s. per week, had been made, he estimates that a saving of about £40 per annum might have been effected to the rates, the cost of hospital treatment in the past two years having been £95 and £270 respectively.

even though in practice it is often remitted, tends seriously to limit the usefulness of the hospital. Charges may, however, be properly made in the case of persons brought from outside the district, or for accommodation of an exceptional character if desired by the patient (see § 16, Isolation Hospitals Act, 1893).

The Royal Commission of 1882 on this point said:

"In favour of the recovery of the expense of hospital treatment is the obvious argument that those who receive what is assumed to be a benefit should pay for it if they can.

"On the other hand the following considerations are not without weight. The person who is thus required to pay for his hospital treatment may have been compelled without any choice of his own or of those in charge of him, or perhaps even against their will, to submit to it. The sanitary authorities will find much difficulty in drawing the line between those who can and those who cannot be fairly expected to pay. It has in point of fact been found almost impossible to exact payment even in cases where it was plainly due. It is desirable in the public interest to attract to these hospitals, even by the bribe of gratuitous treatment, all who will go thither. A payment made by one class for accommodation which is afforded without payment to another, appears to place the latter on the footing of paupers, which it is desirable to avoid. And it is not to be forgotten that the well-to-do persons on whom alone the claim can be made are probably ratepayers who will have contributed more to the maintenance of the hospital than those who will have been treated gratuitously."

In London, admission to the hospitals of the Metropolitan Asylums Board is now free to inhabitants of all classes; see Chapter XVI.

Means of removal. By § 123, Public Health Act, 1875, it is enacted that

> Any local authority may provide and maintain a carriage or carriages suitable for the conveyance of persons suffering under any infectious disorder, and may pay the expense of conveying therein any person so suffering to a hospital or other place of destination[1].

[1] No power appears to be given under the Public Health Acts to local authorities outside London to pay the cost of conveyance back from hospital of persons who have been discharged as cured.

§ 78 of the Public Health (London) Act, 1891, gives similar powers to sanitary authorities in London, and by § 79 the Metropolitan Asylum Managers were empowered to provide and maintain wharves and landing-places for the embarkation and landing of persons removed to or from any hospital belonging to them, and also vessels and carriages suitable for the conveyance of persons suffering from any dangerous infectious disease.

A carriage designed for this purpose is commonly called an "ambulance"—a word which from its etymology would seem to have originally meant a stretcher or litter carried by men walking; but which is now applied in several different senses to arrangements for the care of the sick.

In a Memorandum issued by the Local Government Board in 1876 the following points were mentioned as having to be attended to in the provision and use of ambulances:

1. If the ambulance be intended for journeys of not more than a mile, it may be made so as to be carried between two people, or it may be on wheels and to be drawn by hand. If the distance be above a mile the ambulance should be drawn by a horse. Every ambulance on wheels should have easy carriage springs.

2. In the construction of an ambulance special regard should be had to the fact that after each use it has to be cleansed and disinfected. The entire interior and the bed-frame and bed should be of materials that can be washed.

3. The ambulance should be such that the patient can lie full length in it; and the bed-frame and bed should be movable, so that the patient can be arranged upon the bed before being taken out of his house.

4. With an ambulance there should always be a person specially in charge of the patient; and a horse ambulance should have a seat for such person inside the carriage.

5. After every use of an ambulance for infectious disease it should be cleansed and disinfected to the satisfaction of a medical officer.

6. Both in very populous districts and in districts which are of very wide area, it may often happen that more than one

ambulance will be required at one time; and in any district, if more than one disease is prevailing, there will be an evident advantage in having more than one ambulance for use.

In his *Hospital Report* of 1882 Sir R. Thorne added in amplification of these points: 1st, that it is desirable to have behind the driver's seat a sheet of glass through which an outside attendant may be able to keep the patient in view; 2nd, that

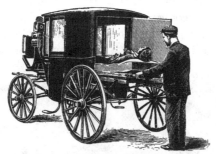

Fig. 24.   Patent Brougham Ambulance[1].

[1] *Description of Patent Brougham Ambulance.*   " Like Ordinary Brougham in appearance, with opaque glass windows at the sides; these window-glasses prevent the public from seeing who is inside, but the patients inside can see outside, thus obviating the use of objectionable curtains.

" Doors at sides and one at back.

" Fitted with portable stretcher which is made with Dominion patent wire mesh and spiral springs; this runs in on a grooved frame which will extend, and then neatly folds up out of the way when not required for the stretcher; the whole of the frame and stretcher can be removed in a minute, then the Ambulance can be used as an ordinary four-seated Brougham should the patients not want to lie down.   The stretcher is fitted with folding handles, and four inside cushions which are covered with rubber sheeting.

" The body is hung on our patent rubber ball bearing springs, patent axles, brake, rubber tyred wheels; the whole arrangement being perfect for ease, and reduces jolting and shaking to a minimum.

" There are two lamps to light the outside, and also one outside lamp to light the inside of body; well ventilated.

" The inside is fitted with a small cupboard for medical accessories.

" It is painted like an ordinary Brougham outside, the inside is finished in self-coloured wood, with four coats of special varnish, which will easily disinfect and wash.

" It is fitted with shafts for one horse, and the whole completed has a pleasing and graceful appearance.

" There is sitting room in the interior for two persons in addition to the patient on stretcher."   This description is taken from the catalogue of Messrs Wilson and Stockall, the makers, Bury, Lancashire.

a box or case containing a stimulant, which it might be necessary to administer during the journey, should be provided in connection with the conveyance; and 3rd, the extreme importance of always placing the ambulance, especially during its journeys from and to the hospital, in charge of a person who can be fully trusted to permit no communication with persons on the route. [It is very desirable that he should be a total abstainer.]

In view of the extreme sensitiveness of public feeling on the subject of the conveyance of infectious patients to hospital through the streets, ambulances are commonly made to resemble in outward appearance a brougham or private omnibus,

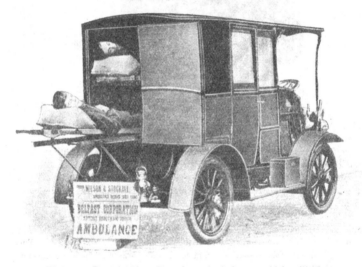

Fig. 25.   Patent Motor Brougham Ambulance, which will close up
like an ordinary Private Brougham[1].

[1] *Description of body of Motor Ambulance.* "Doors at the sides and back, opaque windows, which prevent the patients from being seen from the street, but the patients can see outside.   The best and most up-to-date Ambulance produced—giving speed and safety—for the removal of sick, infectious or accident cases.   Recumbent patients are placed in position through the door at the rear of body.

"Fitted with two stretchers, mounted on small easy springs and wheels, which run in on rabbeted frames, easy and simple to place.   These can easily be removed, either one or both, when not required, the interior of the Ambulance may then be used as an ordinary four-seated Brougham.

"When the stretchers are in use, and in position, there is seating accommodation in the interior for two persons in addition."

with no lettering or mark which might attract attention or cause alarm[1]. (See the annexed illustrations, Figs. 24, 25, 26.)

These figures show ambulances suitable for the removal of infectious cases, made by Wilson and Stockall, Bury, Lancashire.

In recent years two great improvements in the construction of ambulances have been introduced. The first is the substitution for wooden wheels with iron tyres of bicycle wheels with solid rubber, or more recently, pneumatic tyres, by which much smoother running is obtained. The other is the use of the petrol motor for traction in substitution for horse-power, by which the time taken on the journey can be much reduced. These inventions, together with the better condition of the roads in recent years and modern facilities of telephonic communication, have rendered it possible to remove patients to hospital with less fatigue and from much longer distances than was considered practicable at the time of Sir R. Thorne's inquiry[2].

The ambulance is kept in a shed at the hospital, or in the District Council's yard, as local circumstances may render most convenient. It should be disinfected by spraying or otherwise every time between use for one patient and another; and if it is not kept at the hospital, before its removal from the premises. With this view the interior of the vehicle should be metal lined, and all the fittings should be of washable materials. The bed should be of rubber, air filled, with a wire frame, running on rollers, so that it can be pulled out at the back or side.

A nurse usually accompanies the ambulance to take charge of the patient, and at Plaistow Hospital, as mentioned in Chapter XII, she takes notes of the patient's home conditions and of any other infection to which he may have been

---

[1] The proposal of a Town Council to provide by means of loan a vehicle for use, as occasion required, either as an ambulance for conveying patients to the isolation hospital, or as a prison van, did not receive the sanction of the Local Government Board.

[2] In 1911 the average length of journey from the several ambulance stations of the Metropolitan Asylums Board varied from 10·6 to 7·6 miles in the removal of fever patients from their homes to the Board hospitals, and from 26·1 to 40·1 miles in the transfer of convalescents from town to convalescent hospitals. In this year the substitution of motor for horse traction was being carried out but was not completed.

exposed, with a view to his location in the wards[1].   She carries
a case containing milk, water and stimulant jars, with measure

[1] The form used for diphtheria cases is annexed. Similar forms are used for
scarlet fever and enteric fever, but the scarlet fever form contains spaces for notes as to
delirium and desquamation, and the enteric fever form spaces for notes as to epistaxis,
headache, abdominal pain, sputum, rigor, hæmorrhage, supposed cause, milk supply,
etc.

PLAISTOW HOSPITAL, E.

.... 19 ......

PARTICULARS OF CASE OF <u>DIPHTHERIA</u> TO BE TAKEN BY AMBULANCE NURSE

Name in full..

Address ....

Age..................... *M.S.W. Religion*....................... *Occupation* ....

Name and Address of Responsible Person...

Case diagnosed as.................................... *Medical Attendant—Dr*..........................

Date of his last visit................................... *Date illness commenced*......................

Can hair be cut?............................ *Permission given by*..

Vomiting?.. *Sore throat?*......................................

Date, character, and situation of any rash...

Cough?.................................. *If laryngeal, how long?*...

Recession?.............................. *Previous attacks of Croup?*.......................................

Glands enlarged?..

Urine.. *Bowels*...

Ear Discharge—past, present?..

Nasal Discharge—past, present?...

Past illness..

....

Any cases of similar illness in house now or recently?..

Any Antitoxin given? If so, when and how much?..

Any further remarks...

Signed..

To have bath in bed, bathroom.   *Initials of M.O.*...

PARTICULARS TO BE ADDED BY SISTER AFTER ADMISSION

Condition of hair and scalp..

Any injuries, marks, skin disease, etc. ....

....

Any further remarks...

....

Signed..

NOTE.—The above particulars are to be copied into the Ward Report Book.

and feeder for the patient on long journeys; glass receiver and towel in case of sickness; boxes for clean and used swabs to control infective discharges from the mouth and nose; and tongue spatula, taper and matches for examining throats on arrival.   The case is all metal, and any article in it that is wanted can be removed without touching the others. (Biernacki, *Nursing Times*, May 23, 1908.)   The procedure on reception of the patient at the hospital is described in the next chapter.

Effect of removal to hospital on the condition of patients. This is a point on which it is difficult to make any general statement, as the ability of patients to bear removal varies with the nature, severity and stage of the disease from which they

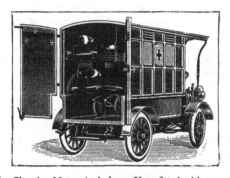

Fig. 26.   Showing Motor Ambulance Van, fitted with two stretchers.

are suffering.   Small-pox patients and convalescents from scarlet fever are often removed without harm over distances of many miles; but cholera patients are said to bear removal badly; removal in the later stages of enteric fever may involve risk of hæmorrhage or perforation of the bowel, and in the later stage of diphtheria, sudden death from failure of the heart. Probably more depends on the careful handling of the patient in getting him from his bed to the ambulance, and from the latter to the ward, than upon the actual distance travelled in a smooth-running ambulance over good roads.

The following report on the effect on patients of removal to hospital was appended to the Annual Report of the Medical Officer of Health for Bristol for the year 1899:

"The Fever Hospital is about four miles from the middle of the city, and the route is along a very hilly road.

"The ambulances are of the Brougham type with solid rubber tyres.

"It was thought at first that there might be some danger in bringing patients this distance during the acute stage of Scarlet Fever, and this question has, therefore, received careful consideration.

"The chief evidence is the comparison between the condition of the patient on his admission and his condition later in the day or on the day following.

"Statistics can scarcely help much, but the temperature charts have all been watched, with a view to finding out whether the condition of the patient was obviously affected by removal.

" Scarlet Fever.

"In about 65 per cent. of cases of Scarlet Fever the temperature on admission was higher than that recorded at any subsequent taking during the uncomplicated stage of the disease.

"This may be due to one of two causes :—either the journey in the ambulance produced a rise of temperature, which subsided with rest in bed, or else the fact that the appearance of the rash—which usually coincides with the height of the disease—is generally the signal for removal to a Fever Hospital.

"That the former is at least a factor is shown by the fact that cases by no means always come in in the height of the disease, and further, some cases which on admission register 103° Fahr. drop that evening, perhaps to 99° Fahr., and do not subsequently rise higher.

"In about 30 per cent. of cases the temperature either continues to rise after admission or else falls at first, to rise higher during the next few days.

"Speaking generally, no case has been actually endangered by removal, though nearly all the severest cases are affected slightly by it, whilst headache and vomiting during transit or on admission, where these symptoms have not been present previously, are occasionally met with.

" Typhoid Fever.

"Cases are not removed after the second week of the disease, if at all severe.

"One patient had slight hæmorrhage for the first time on admission, and several of the severest cases are undoubtedly somewhat exhausted, but no permanent bad effects have been noticed.

"This is evidenced by the fact, that up to the time of writing (May 20), 50 Typhoid patients have been admitted, 49 of which have recovered, and the one death was in no way hastened by the transit.

"Diphtheria.

"In one case death—inevitable anyhow—was probably hastened by the journey, the child dying of cardiac failure about two hours after admission.

"No other patient has been visibly affected by removal.

"F. Percival Mackie, M.R.C.S., L.R.C.P.,

Resident Medical Officer."

In the annual report of Dr J. Brownlee for 1901 on the administration of the City of Glasgow Fever and Small-Pox Hospitals, Belvedere, is a note on the subject of removal to hospital of patients suffering from enteric fever[1]. The medical practitioner or the medical officer of health needs to decide whether the advantage to the patient lies on the side of retaining him at home or removing him to hospital. This point arises particularly when the nature of the disease is not diagnosed until the third week has been reached. In such cases the distance of the hospital is commonly supposed to be an important element in the risk of hæmorrhage or of perforation of the intestine involved in removal. Dr Brownlee has tabulated the number of cases of enteric fever occurring in patients aged 10 years and upwards who have been removed from each mile zone to Belvedere Fever Hospital since the introduction of pneumatic-tyred ambulances, and the corresponding fatality. The numbers in each of the first four zones varied from 441 to 921, a sufficient number to eliminate mistakes due to accidental causes of variation.

In patients admitted from a distance of one mile, the fatality was 21·7 per cent., in patients admitted from a distance of one to two miles it was 20·3 per cent., from a distance of two to three miles it was 21·3 per cent., and from a distance of three to four miles it was 21·1 per cent. In other words, the distance from which the patients were removed made no difference, so far as the prospects of recovery were concerned. This is a valuable result, and it ought to remove prejudices against the removal of enteric patients who cannot be safely and efficiently nursed at home. Dr Brownlee has also investigated the influence of date of removal on the prospects of the patient. His conclusion is that, "though the death-rate among the cases removed to hospital in the third week exceeds that of those removed in the first and second, yet that result is just as likely to be due to the want of attention received during the earlier stage of the fever, where there is often great lack of skill and knowledge of nursing." And it may be added that, as there is great danger of other

[1] Quoted by the late Dr Sykes in his annual report on the health of St Pancras for 1902.

members of the family becoming infected where there is any lack of skill or knowledge in nursing an enteric fever patient, removal to a hospital is strongly indicated.

Risk to the Public through the removal of infectious patients to hospital. The danger of infection to persons in the street or living in houses along the route from the passage of ambulances conveying patients to the hospital is an objection frequently raised by opponents of a hospital scheme. There does not appear, however, to be any evidence that danger to the public arises from the conveyance through the streets of persons suffering from infectious diseases, if effected in a proper ambulance and with ordinary care. The exposure, it must be remembered, is only a momentary one, and it occurs only once in the course of the case, whereas dangerous home conditions will exert their influence during its whole course.

On this point the Hospitals Commission in 1882 reported : " We cannot ignore the fact that a certain amount of risk must be supposed to attach to the passing of ambulances conveying small-pox patients through crowded streets. This danger, however, with proper precautions may probably be reduced to a very small one. No evidence has been brought before us in proof that small-pox prevails in the streets actually traversed by ambulances more than in other streets in the same neighbourhood, and granting a certain possibility of mischief, it remains indispensable for the safety of the whole community that many small-pox patients should be sent away from their homes, and the risk, such as it is, incurred. That ill-managed ambulances propagate disease by the admission of friends into the carriage, by neglect of disinfection, and by loitering at public-houses[1], at the entrance to the hospital and elsewhere, is not only possible, but evident." They gave several recent instances.

---

[1] In the only case known to the writer in which infectious disease was believed to have been contracted from an ambulance, two men in charge of an ambulance conveying a small-pox patient to hospital left it by the roadside while they went into a public-house to drink, and on coming out they found it surrounded by an inquisitive crowd. The men were summoned and fined under § 126, Public Health Act, 1875.

BIBLIOGRAPHY

Copnall. The Law of Infectious diseases and Hospitals. 1899.

Roche. The Telephone and Hospitals for Infectious diseases. Public Health, March, 1896.

Thorne. Hospital Report 1882, and preface to reprint. 1901.

Charges for patients in Isolation Hospitals. Public Health, August, 1897. (Quotes opinion of Mr A. Macmorran, Q.C.)

Mair, L. W. Darra. Report to the Local Government Board on the sanitary circumstances and administration of Gainsborough, with special reference to the prevalence of Fever therein. 1899.

Sweeting, R. D. Report to the Local Government Board on the sanitary condition and administration of the borough of Ilkeston. 1910.

Report of Hospitals Commission. 1882.

Report of Metropolitan Asylums Board. 1911.

Biernacki, J. Modern Fever Nursing. Nursing Times, May, 1908.

Power. Fulham Hospital Report.

Fosbroke, G. H. Removal of patients to Isolation Hospitals. Public Health, Feb. 1895.

Davies, D. S. Annual Report. Bristol, 1899.

CHAPTER XII

MEASURES FOR THE PREVENTION OF CROSS-INFECTION— "BED ISOLATION," OPEN-AIR TREATMENT

THE close aggregation of patients suffering from infectious diseases has long been recognised as detrimental to their own welfare, as well as dangerous to other persons, especially to those in attendance on them.

Thus in former years when typhus fever was the disease especially requiring hospital treatment there were, as we saw in the first chapter, many experienced physicians who considered it better to scatter the typhus cases among other patients in general wards than to collect them into special wards or buildings, holding that the risk of infecting other patients in the first method was a less evil than the danger certain to accrue to the patients themselves and to the staff from the crowding together of typhus patients in wards, then too often ill-ventilated. The danger arising from the aggregation of fever patients was attributed to the concentration of the typhus poison in the air of the wards, and the safeguards recognised were good ventilation, and an ample distance (12 ft.) between patient and patient.

Later, attention was drawn to the apparent increase of activity of the small-pox virus when a number of patients in the acute stage were collected together, as evidenced by the ability to distribute small-pox to persons living in the environs of the hospital, and Sir W. H. Power was inclined to think that this was not merely a matter of concentration of the poison and greater demonstrability of its effects, but that there was under such circumstances an enhanced activity in the strain of the hypothetical infective organism analogous to the increased vigour conferred upon strains of animals and plants by cross-fertilisation.

More recently, when scarlet fever has been the disease most often treated in hospital, on occasions when the wards have been overcrowded ill-effects have appeared to arise, such as increased liability to complications in the course of the disease, and to the occurrence of "return cases" after the patients' discharge. Ill-effects also upon the health of the nurses seemed more liable to occur[1].

But apart from the effects of overcrowding, it has been asserted by opponents of hospital isolation that the mere bringing together of a number of cases such as scarlet fever renders its type more severe, and increases the liability to complications as well as to prolonged infectiveness such as gives rise to return cases. The progressive diminution of the case-mortality of scarlet fever in hospitals, as shown by the Tables on pp. 27 30, is incompatible with the hypothesis of a general or net increase of severity in type—indeed, as already mentioned, it has been cited as evidence of a contrary effect—but obviously the bringing together of a number of patients into one ward, though they may all be supposed to be suffering from the same disease, increases the chance of some other infective or septic organism being present, and the nearer the patients are together

---

[1] It may be noted that a time when a hospital is overcrowded is apt to be for the nurses a time of overwork, curtailment of hours of rest and sleep, irregularity of meals, and lack of exercise in the open air. These things would be likely to impair their health, and render them more liable to contract disease, apart from any greater concentration of poison or enhanced activity of the virus. At such a time, too, precautions in nursing which involve trouble are likely to be relaxed or neglected.

the greater is the opportunity for cross-infection to take place in the absence of special precautions to prevent it.

As already mentioned in Chapter II all isolation hospitals are liable to receive a somewhat large number of patients sent in under an erroneous diagnosis, whose cases prove to be an infectious disease different from that under the name of which they were sent in, or perhaps a disease not infectious at all. Also a patient coming in with one infectious disease may at the same time be incubating or acting as a " carrier " of another. For these reasons the ideal to be aimed at is the isolation of the patient with an infectious disease, not only from susceptible persons outside the hospital, but also, so far as may be necessary to prevent the spread of contagion from other patients in the hospital, even if supposed to be suffering from the same disease[1].

There are several lines along which precautions may be taken against cross-infection. One is the preliminary sorting of cases with a view to preventing those which are of a mixed or doubtful nature, or otherwise a source of possible danger, being placed in the general wards with other patients. At the Plaistow Hospital the system adopted to this end is as follows :

The ambulance nurse when fetching a patient makes full inquiries as to any infection to which he may have been exposed other than that of the disease from which he has been notified as suffering, and as to any diseases from which he may previously have suffered, and the medical superintendent has power to refuse to take in patients whom he cannot isolate with safety to those already under his care. Each case is examined in the ambulance by a

---

[1] " If the child sent to a fever hospital, whether with scarlet fever or diphtheria, can be isolated in his ward to the extent that he is not exposed to infection from his neighbours—either the infection of the disease from which he is not suffering (scarlet fever or diphtheria as the case may be) or the more virulent form of infection of the disease from which he is suffering, which may very well happen under existing circumstances to be communicated to him—a great advance will have been made in securing true isolation in institutions which are now isolation hospitals only in a somewhat limited sense. The existing fever hospital is certainly 'isolation' as far as the great body of the public is concerned, but is in no sense isolation of the sufferer amongst his fellow sufferers." L. Parkes, " The prevention of Diphtheria outbreaks in Hospitals for children," *Public Health*, June, 1903.

Reference may also be made to a very valuable paper, "Some practical points in the management of an isolation hospital," by Dr Knyvett Gordon, medical superintendent of the Monsall Hospital, Manchester, in *Public Health*, March, 1905.

resident medical officer previous to admission to the wards, and upon this examination and the history obtained by the ambulance nurse, the patients admitted fall into three groups, viz. (*a*) those with regular infections which can be placed in a large ward without any special precautions, (*b*) those which can be "barriered" (*i.e.* nursed with special precautions to be presently mentioned) in a large ward, and (*c*) those which must go to a separation ward.

In the location of the patients the information obtained as to the diseases from which they are said to have previously suffered, though not always trustworthy, is found very useful; thus a patient who has been exposed to the infection of a second disease, as for instance measles, can be placed where he will have as his neighbours others who have already had that disease.

At other hospitals the practice is to take the patient to a receiving room where he can be examined and have a bath before being sent to the wards. In this event care is necessary that he shall not be exposed to infection left there by a previous case.

It is desirable in all cases, and especially if there is any doubt, that the patient shall be seen by the doctor as soon as possible after his arrival and before he is placed in a ward with other patients. In small hospitals where there is no resident medical officer, and where there may be some delay before the doctor's visit, the patient should in the meantime be placed in a ward by himself; and the small single-bed wards, which have been already described in Chapter VI, are useful for this purpose. At some hospitals at which post-scarlatinal diphtheria has been very troublesome, it has been found necessary to make a routine practice of taking from the throat of every scarlet fever patient admitted, a swab for examination for the diphtheria bacillus, the patient being kept in a separation ward until the result is known. If the bacillus is found the patient is treated apart from the uncomplicated scarlet fever cases. The adoption of this practice has proved successful in putting an end to the difficulty (Scatterty, "Hospital Isolation," *Public Health*, March, 1905).

The adoption of the above-mentioned practice will generally render unnecessary in all probability the course which has been suggested of giving a prophylactic dose of antitoxin to all children admitted into scarlet fever wards; though possibly such treatment

may be useful where there has been known exposure to diphtheria
infection, or where diphtheria bacilli have been found upon
examination. The prophylactic dose is 500 units, and it confers
protection for two or three weeks. This practice is adopted at
the Pasteur Hospital, Paris.

There is a tendency now to use isolation hospitals for various
other diseases than the three formerly contemplated (scarlet fever,
diphtheria and enteric fever). Thus, it has been usual of late to
isolate serious cases of measles, influenza, cerebrospinal fever,
puerperal fever and in some instances encephalitis lethargica.
It would be costly in construction and expensive in administration
to have separate blocks for each of these diseases. The cubicle
block serves very well for such cases. The cruciform type of
cubicle, with 12 separate cubicles, is a useful one (see figure 48
on page 264).

The following extracts from a report on the working of the
isolation block at Walthamstow (where the "cubicles" are cells,
separated from one another by glass partitions, and entered
directly from the open air) well illustrate the variety of conditions
which may occur at one time requiring separate treatment:

"The cubicle block continues to be of the very greatest value in securing
thoroughly efficient and economical isolation of mixed and doubtful cases."

"In spite of the varied nature of the cases, and the high infectivity of some
of the diseases treated—such as chicken-pox and mumps—no case of infection
being carried from one cubicle to another has occurred."

The following diagram (see next page) shows the cases
actually in the cubicles on June 20th, 1909, and from this the
possibilities of such a ward may be appreciated.

It is taken at random from a number of such records, and
was not specially chosen in any way, except that it was made
when the cubicles were all occupied.

Of the 132 patients treated in the cubicles 18 showed no
definite signs of any infectious disease during their stay in
hospital; 20 were cases of scarlet fever, which had no definite
signs or symptoms on admission, but later showed typical
desquamation; 9 were cases of scarlet fever and diphtheria;
26 were removed to the cubicle block after admission, on account
of suspicious symptoms; the majority of these were patients
admitted as diphtheria, who proved to have no diphtheria

bacilli present, and whose other symptoms suggested that they might have had a slight attack of scarlet fever; 12 were cases of acute nephritis complicating scarlet fever: these are found to make very satisfactory progress in the cubicles, owing probably to the warm equable temperature it is possible to maintain there.

These few particulars may perhaps serve to illustrate what an important part this block plays in the administration of the hospital. It should also be taken into consideration that each

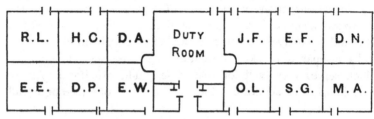

Fig. 27. Diagram of cases treated in the cubicles at Walthamstow Isolation Hospital.

R.L.—Admitted as diphtheria, symptoms suggest scarlet fever only.

H.C.—Is suffering from diphtheria, but has shown some desquamation very suggestive of scarlet fever also.

D.A.—Admitted as diphtheria, proved to be suffering from scarlet fever only; very septic.

J.F.—Scarlet fever, symptoms on admission were suggestive of measles.

E.F.—Scarlet fever; septic; has purulent conjunctivitis.

D.N.—Scarlet fever + diphtheria.

E.E.—Diphtheria, but was convalescent from whooping-cough on admission.

D.P.—Scarlet fever, complicated by acute nephritis.

E.W.—Scarlet fever, complicated by acute nephritis.

O.L.—Scarlet fever + diphtheria.

S.G.—Admitted as scarlet fever; two days after admission developed measles rash.

M.A.—Scarlet fever; other members of family have measles at present.

cubicle can be thoroughly disinfected without any delay and without any inconvenience to any other patients in the block, and that it is not necessary to provide any sick room accommodation for the staff, as any illness, infectious or otherwise, can be satisfactorily dealt with in a cubicle.

It has been already pointed out in Chapter VI that there are several forms of separation wards or cubicles, differing from one another in the completeness of the degree of aerial separation of one bed from another, and that the choice between these forms

will depend largely upon the "striking distance" of the disease
which is under treatment.   If this is spread only by contact
infection or by droplets expelled in coughing and carried through
the air for short distances only, an incomplete screen may suffice,
or it may even be sufficient to carry out careful antiseptic precautions in nursing with no separation other than an ample
space between adjoining beds.   But if the infection is capable of
being wafted through the air for longer distances complete aerial
separation is necessary.

The experience of Dr Caiger with the partially separated
cubicles at the South Western Hospital, Stockwell, as well as that
of Dr Biernacki with "barrier" nursing at the Plaistow Hospital,
go to show that these methods do not suffice, and complete
separation is required in the case of small-pox and chicken-pox,
of measles during the eruptive stage of the disease, and in a less
degree in septic cases of scarlet fever.   On the other hand, the
above-mentioned methods have been found sufficient to prevent
spread to other patients from cases of non-septic scarlet fever,
of measles in the post-eruptive stage, diphtheria, mumps,
whooping-cough, influenza, enteric fever and local contagious
and parasitic affections, except ringworm to which it is stated
desquamating scarlet fever cases are extremely susceptible.

At the South Western Hospital a separate overall is kept
hung up in each cubicle and the nurse puts it on before attending
to the patient, taking it off on leaving the cubicle.   Between
attending to one patient and another she washes her hands in
the lavatory basin provided in the cubicle.   Separate instruments and utensils are provided for each patient and are sterilised
after use.   The regulations in force are set out in detail by
Dr Caiger in the paper already quoted, as follows:

"(1) During the busy hours, when the washing of patients and the treatment
is being carried out, the nurses are to wear no cuffs, and are to keep their sleeves
turned up.

"(2) The overall is to be put on immediately on entering the cubicle, if the
patient, his clothing, or the bedding requires to be touched.   The overall is to be
taken off, and hung on the hook, before leaving the cubicle.   The only occasion
on which the nurse may leave the cubicle wearing the overall is when she takes
the patient to the bathroom, or to the closet, if he be getting up; or when
carrying an utensil to the closet after use by the patient, if he be in bed.   The

overall belonging to one cubicle is never to be worn by the nurse when entering another one.

"(3) When the nurse has finished attending to the patient the hands are to be well rinsed under the spray, *immediately before* leaving the cubicle, and *after* removing the overall.

"(4) Each cubicle is equipped with a bath blanket, bath towel, hand towel, hair brush, comb, small-tooth comb, soap and flannel; and also with a tongue spatula, throat syringe and ear syringe, all of which are kept in the enamelled iron bed locker, and reserved for that patient's sole use. After the doctor has made his round, all spatulas, nozzles, porringers and medicine glasses which have been used are to be collected and removed to the bathroom for sterilisation; afterwards they are to be taken back to the cubicles.

"(5) The same procedure is to be observed in the case of plates, cups, saucers, knives, forks and spoons, which, after use by patients, are to be collected and taken to the ward scullery to be washed up and sterilised. No article is to be put back on the dresser for future use until after it has been through the steriliser.

"(6) In the serving of meals the nurse is to first go round and prepare each patient, by sitting him up in bed, putting on the bib, etc. so that he may be ready to take the food when brought to him. In doing this, she is to put on the overall and rinse her hands in every case. When subsequently handing him his food simply, as also when handing him any other article from outside the cubicle, such as a book, letter or toy, the nurse is not required to put on the overall or to rinse her hands, unless it is necessary for her to touch the patient or the bedclothes.

"(7) When *bathing patients in the bathroom*, each patient is to be taken there separately wrapped in his bath blanket, together with his bath towel. After bathing, the patient is to be taken to the cubicle, wrapped as before in his bath blanket. The water is then run out of the bath, and the inside well rinsed out, and afterwards sponged over with a solution of 1 in 20 carbolic acid, before another patient is brought into the room for bathing.

"(8) When a patient who is getting up *goes to the water closet* the same precautions are to be observed. No two patients are to be allowed to meet in their passage to and from the closets. As in the case of the bathroom, each patient is to be personally conducted there and back again. After use by any patient, the seat of the water closet is to be wiped over with a cloth wrung out of 1 in 20 carbolic lotion, and the closet freely ventilated by opening the window as soon as it has been vacated."

Dr Caiger says:

"In view of the importance we attach to the careful observance of these regulations by the nurses, the reasons underlying them are explained to each nurse at the time she is put to work in the cubicle wards, and it is also impressed upon her that it is on her conscientious attention to the details above enumerated that the success or failure of the treatment will depend. In this way her intelligent interest is enlisted, and her loyal co-operation in the work is likely to be secured. Very careful supervision is exercised by the sister in charge of the ward, and any laxity observed on the part of her subordinates in respect to the technique is severely dealt with."

The procedure at the Walthamstow Hospital is similar, but differs slightly in details. The overalls are hung up in the verandah instead of in the cubicles, and the lavatory basins are also in the verandah instead of in the cubicles, and they are provided with self-closing push-taps which are less expensive than the pedal taps in use at the South Western Hospital. As the nurse washes her hands with disinfecting soap in the basin, after filling it with water, and does not need to touch the taps again, the pedal action is not necessary as it is where she merely rinses her hands in the running spray. On the outside of the door of each occupied compartment hangs a disc, white or red; white if the patient inside has definite and uncomplicated scarlet fever; red if the case is one of doubtful nature or mixed infection. By each door bearing a red disc hangs a separate overall, which the nurse puts on before entering and removes on coming out, washing her hands before going on to the next case. If the disease is uncomplicated scarlet fever it is not considered necessary to put on a separate overall before visiting each patient.

At the Plaistow Hospital the "barriered" cases are distinguished by a coloured cord between two uprights at the foot of the bed. The beds on the left side of the ward in the half nearest the duty room are for ordinary acute cases of the regular infection and have a blue cord. Those on the right side of the same half have a red cord and are for cases in a minor degree dangerous to others, as from slight septic complications or verminous cases, or those who have been in contact with a second infection, but are probably protected by a previous attack. The further end of the ward beyond the entrance to the sanitary annexe, which is in the centre of the side, is for patients who have passed the acute stage, and have no septic lesions or complications. They are not allowed to enter the barriered half of the ward. The nursing of the "barriered" cases is carried out on lines similar to those adopted in the cubicle wards at the South Western Hospital. The nursing appliances and personal articles required by the patient are kept on a shelf and in a locker by his bed for his sole use, and are sterilised after each time of using. The nurse is not allowed to enter the "barriered" space without putting on an overall kept there for her use while attending to the particular patient, and she rinses her hands in a disinfecting solution on each occasion after touching the patient or his surroundings.

The principle of barrier work, according to Dr Biernacki, is to carry on prevention in three zones, one beyond the other. These zones are (*a*) at the source, viz. the point at which the virus is escaping from the body, (*b*) in the immediate neighbourhood of the patient, practically represented by the bed, and (*c*) in the ward at large. Of these, control at the source is to be aimed at, but the common infectious diseases vary greatly as regards the extent to which source-control can be made effective, and in most of them source-control is only partial, so that preventitive measures have to be applied in later stages, to prevent dispersal of the virus. The means of control of infection at the source are classified as "continuous," *e.g.* the catching of infectious discharges from the nose, eyes or ears in pads of boracic wool, and "intermittent," *e.g.* the periodical washing or spraying of those cavities with a disinfectant solution.

Dr Rundle, medical superintendent of the Fazakerley Hospital, Liverpool, goes farther, and maintains that by means of "bed-isolation," *i.e.* a system of nursing precautions less complete than those carried out at the South Western and Plaistow Hospitals, cases even of diseases so infectious as chicken-pox and measles in the first days of eruption may be treated in a ward with other patients without communicating the disease. He states that "41 cases of varicella (chicken-pox) received treatment in the bed-isolation ward; no instance of cross-infection occurred. On the other hand, varicella has been accidentally introduced into the ordinary wards of the hospital on 21 occasions during the same period of time; cross-infection occurred in every instance except one. Precisely the same opportunities for aerial infection were present in each group of cases."

At the Fazakerley Hospital cases of erysipelas, cellulitis and non-infectious disorders are treated with ordinary cleanliness only, no special isolation measures being adopted; but with cases of varicella, pertussis, and doubtful or genuine cases of scarlet fever or diphtheria more rigid measures are taken. Two long coats kept for each case are worn, one by the doctor and the other by the nurse, while examining or attending to the patient. Drinking vessels, knife, fork, spoon and spitting-mug are boiled after use, and separate sanitary utensils, bowl and brush for washing, and bath blankets are reserved for the use of each patient. No interchange of books or toys is permitted. After removing the coat worn in attending to the case the doctor or nurse washes the hands in water containing lysol before proceeding to another case, for which purpose a table with three bowls is kept halfway down each ward. Temperatures are taken in the axilla and the thermometers washed in lysol after use ; a separate one being kept for each patient suffering from varicella or enteric fever. No attempt is made to disinfect the nose or throat nor are oils applied to the skin, except for the prevention of scarring. Care is taken in the location of patients to place those near together which are least likely to be dangerous to one another.

Dr Rundle states that in the two years 1910—11, 741 cases were admitted to the bed-isolation ward suffering from a large variety of diseases, but that in only two cases did cross-infection occur; in both the secondary disease was scarlet fever, in one contracted after rubella which had been notified as scarlet fever, and in the other after diphtheria.

In view of this difference of opinion further observations on the subject are very desirable, but it seems clear that one of the conditions of success in "bed-isolation" is a specially trained staff of nurses, and where this cannot be secured it will be the safer course to continue to treat patients with different infections in wards which are aerially distinct.

In the Medical Supplement to the *Annual Report of the Metropolitan Asylums Board* for 1911, Dr A. F. Cameron gives an account of the treatment of scarlet fever on aseptic lines in the experimental ward at the South Eastern Hospital. The two wards contain 22 beds each, with 2000 c. ft. of space per bed. The fireplace and lavatory are in the centre, between the two ends of the ward, one of which contains 10 beds—five on each side ; and the other 12 beds—six on each side. The admissions were limited to cases of scarlet fever in which the diagnosis had been confirmed in the receiving-room. The section with 10 beds was used for the acute cases, and the 12-bed section for the convalescent cases. The acute cases on admission were placed in the beds nearest the fireplace; and as fresh cases arrived, the older ones were moved towards the end of the ward ; when convalescent they were shifted to the beds nearest to the fireplace in the other section, and moved gradually towards the end, the object being to put the most acute cases in the most convenient position for nursing, and the most convalescent ones at the greatest distance from the acute ones. The method of nursing was similar to that employed in a cubicle block, except that cloaks were not worn.

During the period of 20 months reported on, from April, 1910, to Dec. 31, 1911, 403 scarlet fever patients were treated in these wards during their whole illness in addition to 31 who spent part of their time there, but were transferred for various reasons. Of the 403 cases six died, or 1·5 per cent., and 397 recovered. The patients who recovered spent on an average 42·2 days in hospital, the average residence of all scarlet fever cases in the South Eastern Hospital during 1911 being 47·7 days.

The proportion of complications among the 403 patients so treated was as regards some, as otitis, albuminuria and secondary adenitis, distinctly less than the proportions in the Metropolitan Asylums Board's hospitals generally. The number of alleged infecting cases discharged and sent home was four, of which two were doubtful; the percentage was therefore 1 per cent. on the highest estimate and 0·5 per cent. on the lowest estimate : the corresponding figures for the South Eastern Hospital in 1910 being 3·3, and in 1911, 2·4.

The wards were invaded by other infections on nine occasions, viz. measles four, varicella two, whooping-cough two, and rubella one ; from six of these no spread took place, but further instances occurred after two of the cases of measles (two cases each), and after one of varicella (five cases).

These results, so far as they go, are encouraging and worthy of repetition. Indeed it would appear that in the adoption of a system of bed-isolation, with the aid of separation wards where necessary, lies the best prospect of overcoming the difficulties attaching to the hospital treatment of scarlet fever, such as the liability to cross-infections and to the prolonged infectiveness which gives rise to return cases. What is to be desired is not so much the demonstration that by the employment of a numerous and exceptionally trained staff of nurses a multiplicity of incongruous diseases can be treated without harm in one ward at the same time, but rather a method within the competence of an ordinary staff of nurses by which such risks of cross-infection and septic complication as attach to the treatment in one ward of a number of cases of the same infectious disease can be avoided.

One essential precaution for the prevention of cross-infection is the maintenance between bed and bed of such a distance as will prevent not only direct contact between the two patients, but also that the one patient shall be out of reach of noxious exhalations and droplets of infectious secretion expelled from the throat and respiratory passages of the other. This distance should not be less than 12 ft., and in some hospitals in certain cases as much as 15 ft. has been allowed.

It is desirable for several reasons that convalescent patients, especially scarlet fever patients, should not remain in the same wards with the acute cases up to the period of their discharge, but that the latter part of their stay, when they are able to get up and move about, though still not clear of infection, should be spent in a separate convalescent ward. This may be planned on cheaper lines than the ordinary ward blocks; it may be a two-storey building with day-rooms on the ground floor and dormitories on the first floor, and the amount of space per bed in the latter need not be so great as in the wards. Day-rooms for convalescents are useful, as already mentioned, but the mixing together of convalescents requires supervision as those with septic discharges are apt to be a danger to others.

Free ventilation of the wards is of obvious importance, both for the well-doing of the patients themselves and to prevent the concentration of poisonous exhalations; the contracting of infection largely depending upon a dosage sufficient to overcome the powers of resistance of the person exposed. The modern view that ventilation is a matter of the temperature, degree of humidity and movement of the air rather than of the replacement of fouled air by pure air is not applicable to hospitals for infectious diseases, where the question is not one only of chemical impurities but also of pathological products and pathogenic bacteria. Dr J. S. Haldane, F.R.S., while setting forth the views above referred to says, " It seems to me there are clear reasons for demanding a far higher standard of ventilation in rooms where the risk of infection through the air appears to be specially great."

It is maintained by some physicians that not only cases of pulmonary tuberculosis, but even those of acute infectious diseases may advantageously be treated as nearly as possible in the open air, with the protection merely of a roof to keep off rain. This system has been carried out for several years by Dr Boobbyer at the Bagthorpe Hospital, Nottingham. It was adopted with a view of overcoming the disadvantages attendant upon the aggregation of patients suffering from acute specific diseases, especially scarlet fever, of all types in large common wards. At first schemes were considered for providing small separate wards, one for each case, but these were abandoned as impracticable. He then augmented the ventilation of the wards by open windows, and the advantage was at once apparent in the improved health of the staff and patients. Finding that this free ventilation was well borne even by acute and severe cases[1], but that it did not altogether do away with cross-infection so long as the patients were treated in the wards, he began to treat acute and severe cases of scarlet fever and small-pox in the open air, and this practice has been regularly followed since 1899, with, it is said, excellent results. Dr Boobbyer says :

[1] Miss Nightingale says, " In the wooden hospital huts before Sebastopol with their pervious walls and open ridge ventilators, in which the patients sometimes said that they would get less snow if they were outside, such a thing as 'catching cold' was never heard of. The patients were well covered with blankets, and were all the better for the cold air."

"Cases of small-pox, scarlet fever, measles, whooping-cough, pneumonia, erysipelas, and even enteric fever have been nursed under these open-air conditions, without untoward result in any single instance. Speaking generally, septic cases clear up much more speedily under such conditions than when confined to the wards. Neither pneumonia nor bronchitis has developed in any instance, and even nephritis cases have improved more rapidly than when nursed inside the wards.

"In 1901, owing to the success which had attended our long continued experiment with open-air treatment for all classes of cases, and the disquieting frequency of cross-infection among the cases of different diseases nursed in our isolation block, and of hospital throats among the staff, I advised the health committee to convert the latter block into an open-air pavilion, with external verandahs. This advice was followed in 1903, and cross-infection in this ward-block has been almost unknown since that date. When the conversion was first carried out, the sisters and nurses of the hospital protested strongly against the exposure involved (to the staff) in nursing a pavilion under these conditions, and assured me that no nurses would undertake the duty in winter time. This prediction has been entirely falsified by subsequent experience, for there is now no section of the hospital so popular with the nurses as the isolation block. I should perhaps explain that sail-cloth curtains are used to protect the verandahs in very bad weather, as with high wind, driving rain and snow, the latter could not be occupied without such protection.

"When patients are first brought under these open-air conditions, it is, of course, desirable to provide them with plenty of covering in the shape of blankets, and if there be much wind to fasten the bed coverings to the bed-stead, and, further, in many instances, at the outset at any rate, to warm the bed with hot bottles; but one of the most remarkable circumstances connected with the treatment is the ease and rapidity with which all sorts of patients, and especially the young, establish a complete tolerance of open-air conditions at all seasons of the year. Patients, moreover, nursed outside during the acute stage of their attack and then taken inside, frequently complain that the internal atmosphere appears close and oppressive, and depressing to their vitality and their spirits.

The results of the open-air treatment of scarlet fever are not very evident statistically. Scarlet fever mortality has diminished in Nottingham as elsewhere—see Table on p. 27—but the case mortality in hospital, though it has diminished among hospital cases since 1899, has diminished still more among home treated ones.

Average annual mortality per 100 cases of scarlet fever.

	7 years (1892—8)		12 years (1899—1910)
Hospital treated......	3·7	...	2·1
Home treated	9·5	...	2·1

The percentage of "return cases" of scarlet fever per 100 convalescents discharged has on the whole diminished somewhat since the adoption of the open-air treatment in 1899, having been 3·9 in the seven years 1892—8, and 2·6 in the 12 years 1899—1910, but it fluctuates too much from year to year for much importance to be attached to the difference. The records of cases, so far as the figures are comparable, do not show any progressive diminution in the frequency of the various complications of scarlet fever, nor on the other hand do they show any increase in the frequency of those which may be thought of as specially likely to be produced by exposure to cold and damp, as nephritis, rheumatism and bronchitis. The open-air treatment of acute and septic cases must at all events remove sources of danger from the patients who are left in the wards, and as it appears when carefully carried out to involve no undue risk to the patients nor difficulty to the staff, it is worthy of trial in appropriate cases in other hands.

The real open-air treatment of scarlet fever could be carried out in a specially built verandah-ward, open in front except for a low wall. A canvas screen could be interposed in case of very strong winds or driving rain; the space between bed centres to be 12 feet. Experience has shown that cases of infectious disease can be treated under such conditions without fear.

Eucalyptus treatment of scarlet fever. In a previous chapter (p. 55) mention has been made of the claim made by Dr R. Milne that by the treatment from the outset of scarlet fever cases with inunction of eucalyptus oil over the skin and swabbing the throat with carbolic oil, the infective nature of the disease can be so counteracted that the necessity for isolation is abolished. The condition postulated by Dr Milne as essential to success—namely that the treatment shall be carried out from the very first commencement of the illness—cannot be complied with in the class of cases that are sent into fever hospitals, as these are usually not admitted until after they have been ill at least one or two days. It has however been assumed that if there is any virtue in the treatment it should be useful in scarlet fever wards in preventing cross-infection and complications, and in preventing patients erroneously sent in as suffering from scarlet fever from contracting the disease in the ward, and in reducing the liability to production of return cases by convalescents on discharge.

As already mentioned in Chapter III, a trial of the treatment by Dr Biernacki at the Plaistow Hospital did not bear out any such expectations, but it is only fair to say that claims of this kind do not appear to have been ever made by Dr Milne himself. The results of a year's experience of the eucalyptus treatment at the South Eastern Hospital, reported on by Dr F. M. Turner in the *Medical Supplement to the Annual Report of the Metropolitan Asylums Board for* 1911, are somewhat less unfavourable.

Into a 20-bed ward (1 A) Dr Turner sent all the doubtful cases, such as had formerly been kept isolated in single rooms. Many of these turned out to be true scarlet fever; others were discharged without, as far as could be ascertained, having had scarlet fever. In addition he freely admitted ordinary unselected cases of scarlet fever. The patients were treated according to Dr Milne's recommendations; when up they played together and mixed in every way usual to children in a large ward. In this ward there were treated during 12 months 201 patients, of whom 141 were certain cases of scarlet fever, 20 were doubtful but probably mild cases of scarlet fever, and 40 were not scarlet fever. In another ward (1 B) were similarly treated 126 cases of whom 105 were certain cases of scarlet fever, 7 were doubtful, and 14 were not scarlet fever. The eucalyptus treatment was also used in some cases of secondary scarlet fever which appeared in the diphtheria wards. The results are given by Dr Turner as follows:

"According to Dr Milne the non-scarlet patients in wards 1 A and 1 B should have been protected against infection, and also the diphtheria cases in such wards as had one or more scarlet cases in them. Also the individual scarlet fever cases should have been free from infection in ten days, if not sooner; consequently no return cases should have arisen in their homes after their discharge however early this had taken place. These predictions were not verified by experience; but on the other hand the prevalent views as to the infectivity of scarlet fever would have led most expert critics to prophesy a very large amount of infection to take place among those exposed, even if all did not contract the disease. The facts were further from this expectation than from the other."

In one case a child with erythema, which had been certified as scarlet fever, was 13 days in the ward with oiled scarlet fever patients without contracting the latter disease, though he was proved to be susceptible to it by getting it from another source two months after his discharge.

In another instance a child in the diphtheria ward who had been attacked by secondary scarlet fever, and had been oiled from the first, remained for two and a half months in the ward with 13 other children of ages one to seven years; only one of these children contracted scarlet fever and that after a month's exposure. The last-mentioned child, however, although oiled, gave scarlet fever to four others.

From these instances Dr Turner concludes that the treatment confers a certain degree of immunity but that the protection is not complete.

Into the scarlet fever wards 1 A and 1 B there were admitted 330 patients of whom 57 were believed not to have had scarlet fever on admission; of these six contracted the disease or 10·5 per cent. On the average of the three preceding years the corresponding proportion among cases treated by the older method of isolation in single rooms was 6·5 per cent.

The number of scarlet fever cases discharged, including doubtful cases, was 226, and following their discharge 10 outbreaks of scarlet fever were reported in the houses to which they went—an infectivity rate of 4·4 per cent. The corresponding infectivity rate at this hospital during the four previous years had been 4·0 per cent. There was therefore no reduction in the proportion of return cases, after the adoption of the eucalyptus treatment, but there was no definite increase although some of the cases had been sent out much sooner than they would have been in previous years. The average detention of all the scarlet fever cases, including doubtfuls, was 44·5 days, or excluding doubtfuls, 45·8 days. In 1909 the average detention of all scarlet fever cases including doubtfuls was 57·4 days.

The treatment appeared to have no effect upon the frequency of complications, one way or the other. Slight albuminuria occurred in 15 per cent. of the cases, and otitis in 13·2 per cent. —these proportions are rather higher than usual, but this is accounted for by the young average age of the children treated.

The cost of eucalyptus oil was £11. No extra nurses were employed. There was a large saving from the shorter stay in hospital which was deemed permissible.

BIBLIOGRAPHY

Murchison, C. A treatise on the continued Fevers of Great Britain. 1873.

Bristowe and Holmes. The Hospitals of the United Kingdom. 1863.

Power. Fulham Hospital Report.

Thorne. Hospital Report. 1882.

Parsons. Hospital Report. 1912.

Marriott, E. D. Scarlet Fever ; the case against Hospital Isolation. 1899.

Millard, C. K. The influence of Hospital Isolation on Scarlet Fever. Public Health, Feb., 1901.

Parkes, L. C. The prevention of Diphtheria attacks in Hospitals for children. Public Health, June, 1903.

Gordon, A. Knyvett. Some practical points in the management of an isolation hospital. Public Health, March, 1905.

Biernacki, J. Modern Fever Nursing. Nursing Times, 1908.

Scatterty. Hospital Isolation. Public Health, March, 1905.

Gellatly, Jessie. In Annual Report of M.O.H. for Walthamstow. 1909.

Caiger, F. F. Cubicle Isolation. Public Health, June, 1911.

Rundle. Proceedings of Epidemiological Section, Royal Society of Medicine. May, 1912.

Rundle and Burton. Lancet, March 16, 1912.

Cameron, A. F. The treatment of Scarlet Fever on aseptic lines. Report of Metropolitan Asylums Board. 1911.

Nightingale, Florence. Notes on Hospitals. 1863.

Haldane, J. S. Standards of Ventilation. Public Health, Oct., 1904.

Hill, Leonard. The physiological basis of the claims for fresh air and ventilation. Public Health, March, 1913.

Boobbyer, P. The open-air treatment of acute infectious diseases. Public Health, May, 1911.

Lauder. Lancet, March 12, 1904.

Chapin, C. V. The importance of contact infection. American Journal of Public Hygiene, Vol. xx. Aug. 1910.

Anderson, A. Scarlet Fever ; some points in the prevention of hospital complications and return cases. Public Health, March, 1905.

Klein, E. Reports on bacteriology of Scarlet Fever in Reports of Medical Officer, Local Government Board. 1885—8.

—— Preliminary Report on the microbes associated with Scarlatina. Report of Medical Officer, Local Government Board. 1896—7.

—— Further Report on Scarlatina. 1897—8.

Gordon, Mervyn. Further reports on the Bacteriology of Scarlatina in Reports of Medical Officer, Local Government Board. 1899—1900 and 1900—1.

—— Report on the fermentative characters of Streptococci present in the fauces during Scarlet Fever. Report of the Medical Officer, Local Government Board. 1910—11.

Jacques, W. K.   The microscope in the diagnosis of Scarlet Fever.   Public Health, Feb., 1903.

Harris, A.   Scarlet Fever from a public health point of view with some investigation into its bacteriology.   Public Health, Sept., 1904.

Prichard, R.   Influence of Ventilation on the type of disease.   Public Health, April, 1903.

Milne, R.   Proceedings of the Epidemiological Section, Royal Society of Medicine.   1909—10.

Turner, F. M.   Report on one year's experience of Dr Milne's inunction treatment of Scarlet Fever.   Report of Metropolitan Asylums Board 1911.

Higgins, T. S.   The Bacillus Diphtheriæ in relation to Return cases of Scarlet Fever.   Public Health, April, 1912.

Millard, C. K.   The Eucalyptus inunction treatment of Scarlet Fever. Public Health, August, 1911.

Ritchie, J.   Diphtheria Carriers and Post-scarlatinal Diphtheria.   Ibid.

Laird, A. J.   Treatment of Scarlet Fever by Eucalyptus Oil.   Public Health, Feb., 1912.

Crookshank, F. G.   The control of Scarlet Fever.   Proceedings of the Epidemiological Section, Royal Society of Medicine.   Jan., 1910

CHAPTER XIII

DISCHARGE OF PATIENTS FROM HOSPITAL

THE discharging from hospital of patients convalescent after an infectious disease is a matter which requires much care and judgment on the part of the medical superintendent. The object of an isolation hospital is frustrated if patients are sent home while still in an infectious state; but on the other hand to detain them longer than is necessary for their recovery and for the cessation of infection is irksome to them, involves unnecessary expense, and occupies space which may be wanted for other cases. The difficulty arises from the fact that, as already mentioned, in certain diseases, as scarlet fever, diphtheria, and enteric fever, infectiousness is apt to persist, or perhaps recur, long after the apparent recovery of the patient, who thus becomes a "carrier," and is liable to give rise to "return cases" after he has returned home. In small-pox this difficulty does not occur, and when the patient feels well enough, and his skin is clear of scabs, he may be safely released after a thorough bathing, cleansing and change of apparel.

In *enteric fever* the long course and debilitating effect of the disease, its liability to accidents and slow convalescence, often necessitate a long stay in hospital[1], but, when the patient is well enough to be discharged, it is not usually necessary to detain him, lest he should be dangerous to others. But in a certain small proportion of cases, estimated at about 2 or 3 per cent., and most frequently in women, virulent typhoid bacilli persist in the intestines, gall bladder or urinary organs for years after recovery, and are voided continuously or intermittently. Such " typhoid carriers " are a continual source of danger, especially if the nature of their vocation involves the handling of food, as in milking, cooking, etc. Hence before a person of any such calling, convalescent from enteric fever, is discharged from hospital it will be well to have a bacteriological examination made of the excretions, and repeated if necessary, in order to ascertain whether the bacilli are still present. They may disappear in the course of a few months, but, should they still persist, no means of getting rid of them is at present known, and it is useless to detain the patient in hospital. The only thing which can be done is to warn him, or her, of the danger, to inculcate habits of extreme cleanliness, especially as regards washing the hands after visiting the closet and before handling food, and to advise if necessary a change of occupation, choosing if possible one in which danger to others will not be incurred.

In diphtheria, in view of the liability to heart failure and to paralyses in the later course of the disease, the interests of the patient forbid a discharge before complete convalescence. When he is well enough to go out, if the mucous membranes of the throat and nose are normal and swabs on examination show no diphtheria bacilli, he may be discharged. It may be necessary to take swabs from the nose as well as the throat, and to repeat the examination after a week's interval if the first is negative, but it does not appear that there is much advantage in requiring

[1] In the M.A.B. hospitals in 1911 the average length of stay of recovered cases of enteric fever was 61·7 days.

a third negative result before discharge[1]. If Klebs-Löffler bacilli are found to be present the case must be retained longer under treatment and further swabs taken, but it is a question

[1] Dr Thomas W. Salmon, Assistant Surgeon U.S. Public Health and Marine Hospital Service, from a study of a series of 100 cases of diphtheria in the Willard State Hospital, New York, gives the following table showing the number of persons out of the hundred who would still have been infectious on discharge according to different methods of release.

After time limit of two weeks (? from onset)	60
After time limit of three weeks ,, ...	37
After time limit of four weeks ,, ...	27
After one negative culture	54
After two negative cultures	13
After three negative cultures	11
After one negative culture after two weeks (from onset)	26
After two negative cultures after two weeks ,,	6
After three negative cultures after two weeks ,,	5
After three negative cultures after three weeks	2
After three negative cultures after four weeks	2

He concludes that

1.   The severity of the disease has no relation to the duration of infection.

2.   Proof is afforded of the unfairness of an arbitrary time limit in the quarantine of diphtheria.

3.   The occurrence of positive cultures after a single negative is shown to be the rule rather than the exception.

4.   The importance of taking cultures from the nose as well as the throat for the release of pharyngeal cases is demonstrated by the number of cases in which the nose remained longer infected.

5.   Two negative cultures taken on alternate days from both nose and throat after two weeks have elapsed from the onset of the disease is suggested as a requirement which is not unfair to any, and which permits the release of only 6 per cent. of infected persons.

Dr W. Hill, Director of Boston Board of Health Bacteriological Laboratory, says that " Release on one negative culture allows 30 per cent. of the total persons released to go out of isolation while bacilli are still present.   A negative culture for release is less reliable than a negative culture for diagnosis, because the bacilli are then fewer, have become scattered, and lie in the folds and follicles of the mucous membrane." Extensive investigation has shown that if two consecutive negative cultures for release be demanded, only 1 to 3 per cent. of those released will be still infective.   To make sure of this 1 to 3 per cent. by requiring three consecutive cultures for release would involve so much additional trouble for the physician and the patient that hitherto it has proved impracticable outside of hospitals.

Dr D. Stewart (*Public Health*, March, 1913) does not find that the system of requiring two negative swabs before discharge has prevented the occurrence of return cases, and has obtained equally good results when patients who were clinically fit for discharge were sent out without ascertaining whether or not they carried the diphtheria bacillus.

whether very long retention in hospital after apparent recovery is advisable, as the bacilli, though present, may have lost their virulence. Cases have occurred in which diphtheria bacilli have persisted in the throat of a person detained for many months in hospital, but inoculation into rodents has ultimately shown them to be non-virulent and the discharge of the patient has been followed by no return cases.

In the Metropolitan Asylums Board's hospitals in 1911 the average stay of diphtheria patients (not merely "bacteriological") who completed their recovery in town hospitals was 58·6 days, and in those transferred to convalescent hospitals 73·6 days. Of cases of "bacteriological diphtheria" the average stay was 27·7 days.

In 1920 it appears to have become the practice at the hospitals of the Metropolitan Asylums Board not to detain carriers of diphtheria beyond a short period after the disappearance of the clinical symptoms of the disease, and they were discharged without waiting for bacteriological evidence that the specific organism was absent from successive throat swabs. While admitting that B. diphtheriæ may lurk for a long time in the throats of certain convalescents, it has been found that in most instances the infectivity of such carriers is not great, and that their discharge from hospital has not so far been attended with untoward results.

It is in connection with the discharge of scarlet fever convalescents that "return outbreaks" at the patient's home and complaints of premature discharge are most frequent. In a person who has had scarlet fever an infective condition may persist or recur during a period of several weeks after apparently complete recovery, and on the convalescent's return to his family, if it includes susceptible persons, other cases, commonly called "return cases," are liable to occur. See Chapter II, p. 33. There do not appear however to be "chronic carriers" of scarlet fever as there are of enteric fever and diphtheria, who may continue infectious for many months or years. In 1176 return outbreaks of scarlet fever classified by Dr Turner[1], the greatest number on any one day, 103, commenced on the 5th day after the convalescent's return, and 441 or 37·5 per cent. in the 1st week; in the 6th week the number had declined to an average of less than 2 per diem,

[1] *Public Health*, April, 1901.

and in the 10th week there was only one outbreak. A certain number of these outbreaks may be due to independent causes, apart from the return of the convalescent, or to the bringing into use on his return of clothing or toys which had been put away without proper disinfection, but Dr Turner only estimates the number of cases which can be so accounted for as 10 per cent., though others have put it higher.

The usual proportion of return cases to 100 scarlet fever convalescents discharged is from 2 to 3·5; the following percentages have been recorded:

Glasgow (Chalmers), 1894	... ...	2·6
Birmingham (Millard), 1896—7 ...	...	3·4
Nottingham (Boobbyer), 1897—9	...	2·2
M.A.B. hospitals (Simpson), 1898—9 ...		2·9
Brighton (Newsholme), 1901	... ...	3·4[1]
Southampton (Lauder), 6 years, ?1904—9		1·9

These proportions may be compared with the 5·6 per cent. of secondary cases after home isolation recorded by Dr Chapin. (See footnote to p. 46, Chapter III.)

Much reliance, however, cannot be placed on percentages of "return cases," unless based on large figures extending over a series of years, for where the numbers are small the rate fluctuates greatly from year to year. Return cases are most numerous at times when the hospital is full, that is usually during an epidemic. It may be that this is because at such times the disease has naturally a greater tendency to spread, owing to an increased virulence of the contagion, to a diminished average power of resistance in the community, or to a large proportion of its members being unprotected by a previous attack, so that the disease is reproduced by smaller doses of infection than would be required at other times. Or it may be that owing to the pressure on the hospital administration at such times, regulations are apt to be relaxed, and overcrowding is liable to occur.

There is also a difference in practice at different hospitals as to the period after the convalescent's return within which further cases that may occur are reckoned as "return cases." The Society of Medical Officers of Health have suggested that the term should

---

[1] *Public Health*, February, 1903.

include cases occurring in the same house or elsewhere, and apparently traceable to the person released within a period of not less than 24 hours, or not more than 28 days after his return or release from isolation. Others have considered that there should be no time limit, but Dr Turner's figures already quoted show that the greater number of farther attacks occur within the first few weeks, and those occurring after a long interval are more likely to be due to an independent source of infection.

The percentage of "infecting cases" is somewhat smaller than that of "return cases," as one infecting case may give rise to more than one "return case." Dr Turner gives the number of "infecting cases" in return outbreaks connected with the Metropolitan Asylums Board's hospitals in the three years 1902—4 as 1262 and of the "infected cases" as 1442. The infecting cases were 3·22 per cent. of the total scarlet fever cases discharged against 1·1 per cent. of the total diphtheria cases discharged. There were also among the "return outbreaks" a number of cross-infections where a diphtheria case had followed the return of a scarlet fever convalescent or *vice versâ*. Among the total 1573 return outbreaks there were 1176 of scarlet fever after scarlet fever, 168 of diphtheria after diphtheria, 101 of diphtheria after scarlet fever, and 44 of scarlet fever after diphtheria, the remainder being cases where the diagnosis was not confirmed or the outbreak could not be traced. The crowding of the crossed cases, as of the others, into the first three or four weeks after the convalescent's return indicated that the majority were really "return cases" and not merely coincidences. Cases both of scarlet fever and diphtheria followed the discharge of a scarlet fever patient in 12 instances, and the discharge of a diphtheria patient in five instances. Adding these, the diphtheria return outbreaks after scarlet fever were 0·32 per cent. of the total scarlet fever discharges and the scarlet fever return outbreaks after diphtheria were 0·32 per cent. of the total diphtheria discharges, an exactly similar proportion. The proportion of infecting cases was less among patients discharged from the convalescent hospitals than among those discharged direct from the acute wards, being 3·75 per cent. in the latter and 2·01 per cent. in the former. The proportion of infecting cases was higher among patients who had been in hospital 8—12 weeks than in those in hospital for shorter periods, and the highest rates occurred in those hospitals which were most consistent in detaining cases until peeling was complete.

Medical opinion formerly considered that the cause of the prolonged infectiousness of scarlet fever was the desquamation from the skin, and this is still the popular belief; but the opinion of medical superintendents at the present time appears to be unanimous that the later desquamation and the peeling of the thick epidermis of the hands and feet may safely be disregarded, and that the seat of infection is to be found in unhealthy conditions of the throat and discharges from the mucous membranes of the nose and ears. Such discharges have been found in a large proportion of infecting cases, and it has been observed that scarlet fever convalescents who had not infected other persons before have done so after contracting a catarrh. Possibly the specific organism lurks in the recesses of the nose and throat, and finds in the catarrhal discharge a suitable medium in which to multiply.

Unfortunately bacteriological tests for infection are not available in scarlet fever, for though various organisms have from time to time been found associated with it, none is as yet established as its cause in the sense that the Bacillus diphtheriæ of Klebs and Löffler is of diphtheria or as the bacillus typhosus of Eberth is of enteric fever; nor is there any easy or certain test for their detection.

It seems, however, to be fairly clear that severe and complicated cases of scarlet fever owe their character to the association—along with the specific organism of scarlet fever—of septic organisms such as the Streptococcus pyogenes, a common causal organism of suppuration, and it may be that septic complications also tend to prolong the stage of infectiousness. There are, however, infecting cases in which no abnormal appearance is to be found.

At the hospitals of the Metropolitan Asylums Board in 1911 the average length of residence of recovered scarlet fever patients treated in town hospitals only was 57·9 days, and of those transferred to convalescent hospitals for completion of their treatment 63·5 days altogether. (The latter would presumably include the more severe and complicated cases.) These figures were 4·8 and 2·0 days respectively below the averages for the preceding ten years. In 1901, following Prof. Simpson's investigation, there had been a reduction of about a week as compared with previous practice. The period of detention at the Metropolitan Asylums

Board's hospitals is longer than that at some other hospitals. The following figures are given by Dr Bond in *Public Health*, Feb., 1903 :

London Fever Hospital.   Minimum detention 6 weeks for adult, had been reduced from 7 weeks to 6 weeks for ages 10— 14, and from 8 weeks to 7 weeks for children under 10 years.

Leicester, 1895.   6 weeks in hospital, or 5 weeks for patients treated with eucalyptus oil.   In 1901 reduced to minimum of 4 weeks in hospital.   Average stay 39·1 days from onset or 35·3 days from admission.

Edinburgh.   Ordinary cases 6 weeks, special cases 7—8 weeks.

Nottingham.   5 weeks or sometimes a month from onset.

Liverpool.   Average 8 weeks.

In no instance had ill effects been observed from the shorter period.

In a report appended to the *Annual Report of the Metropolitan Asylums Board for* 1910, the late Dr H. E. Cuff gave the following figures of the average length of stay of scarlet fever patients in the larger fever hospitals of England and Scotland :

Leeds City Hospital	63 days.
Liverpool City Hospital	7—8 weeks.
Belvedere Hospital, Glasgow	55·3 days (including fatal cases).
Ruchill Hospital, Glasgow	54·4 days.
Edinburgh City Hospital	48·6 days.
Monsall Hospital, Manchester	56 days.

At Huddersfield the period of detention had been reduced to 29 days with a coincident fall in the "return case" rate.

At Southampton during the past six years it had averaged only 30 days and the "return case" rate had been only 1·9 per cent.

(At Southampton the convalescent cases, after a bath and change of clothes as if for discharge, are transferred to a convalescent ward for the last two or three weeks of their stay in hospital. *Lancet*, March 12, 1904.)

As regards the prevention of "return outbreaks" it appears from what has been said that when scarlet fever convalescents feel well enough to go out, and if they are free from discharges from the nose and ears, and the throat is in a normal condition, there is no advantage, but the reverse, in keeping them in hospital until the peeling of the skin is completed. More is to be hoped from the "bed-isolation" of severe and complicated cases, either in separate wards, or by aseptic nursing as mentioned in the last chapter, and by transferring the patient to a separate convalescent hospital for the last week or two of his residence.

Before being discharged the convalescent should have a warm bath, using an antiseptic soap, and including the washing of the hair. If the peeling of the skin of the feet or hands is not completed it may be well, in order to avoid scruple, to paint them with tincture of iodine (especially between the toes) or wrap them in rags soaked in a disinfecting solution. As the patient may "catch cold" if exposed to a low temperature immediately after a hot bath, and the secretion from the nose may be infectious, it is better if possible to keep him for a night after his final bath in a room free from infection before he is discharged from hospital.

The patient will of course have been carefully examined beforehand by the medical officer as to his fitness for discharge both from the clinical point of view and as to the freedom from conditions likely to be infectious. Care should also be taken to see that the head is free from vermin.

But since in the present state of knowledge there are no means of ascertaining that infection has entirely ceased, it will be well that the patient or his relatives should be warned that this is so, and should be advised to take further precautions on his return home. If desquamation has not entirely ceased, this should be noted with an explanation that it need not be regarded as infectious.

It has been recommended by the Society of Medical Officers of Health[1] that notification of the discharge of a fever patient from hospital should be previously sent to the Medical Officer of Health of the district concerned (where he is not himself in charge of the hospital), and that he should also be notified of any errors of diagnosis in cases sent to hospital.

[1] *Public Health*, February, 1903.

By way of example we may quote the following notice sent at Coventry to the parents of every scarlet fever patient before he leaves the City Hospital (*Public Health*, Sept., 1906):

> Every effort is made to ensure that the children are free from infection when discharged from the Hospital, but it is exceedingly difficult to be quite sure of this; parents are therefore urged in cases of scarlet fever to observe the following precautions:
>
> Whenever it is possible the child should be sent for a short time to a house where there are no children, that when this cannot be done, care should be taken that the child does not kiss the other children of the family or come into close contact with them so far as this can be prevented. The child should on no account be allowed to sleep with the others, as this is particularly dangerous.
>
> A bath must be given every night, carbolic soap being used.
>
> Discharges from the ears and nose are very infectious, and if discovered to exist advice should at once be sought from the medical attendant or at the City Hospital.
>
> The child should be taken into the fresh air as much as possible, but must not be sent to school or into any other assembly of children for at least a fortnight.

As regards the powers of the local authority to detain in hospital patients who are not fit for discharge, reference may be made to Chapter XI.

BIBLIOGRAPHY

Report of Metropolitan Asylums Board. 1911.

Ledingham and Th. Thomson. Report on the Enteric Fever "carrier," being a review of current knowledge on the subject. Report of the Medical Officer, Local Government Board. 1909—10.

Gresswell, D. A. On Diphtheria as a chronic malady. Transactions of Epidemiological Society. 1886.

Erskine, A. M. Epidemic Diphtheria. Public Health, Sept., 1904.

Salmon, T. W. Release from Isolation after Diphtheria. Public Health, Jan., 1908.

Hill, W. W. Ibid.

Stewart, D. Duration of Infectivity in Diphtheria. Public Health, March, 1913.

Turner, J. S. Return cases of Scarlet Fever and Diphtheria. Public Health, Oct., 1906.

Thompson, T. W. Report on the re-invasion by Scarlatina of households to which persons from the Bromley and Beckenham Joint Hospital had returned on their recovery from that disease. In Report of Medical Officer, Local Government Board. 1894—5.

Public Health, April, 1901.

Simpson, W. J. Return cases of Scarlet Fever and Diphtheria. Report to Metropolitan Asylums Board. 1901.

Cameron. Ibid.

Bond, F. A. Infectious diseases ; length of stay of patients in hospital and "return cases." Public Health, Feb., 1903.

Cuff, H. E. In Report of Metropolitan Asylums Board. 1910. (Gives figures of length of stay of scarlet fever patients at different hospitals.)

Klein and M. Gordon. See bibliography to Chapter XII.

Mason, J. W. Secondary and Return cases of Scarlet Fever. Public Health, April, 1898.

Fitzsimmon, J. B. Influence of Hospital Isolation on Scarlet Fever in Hereford. Public Health, March, 1903.

Anderson, A. Scarlet Fever ; some points in the prevention of hospital complications and return cases. Public Health, March, 1905.

Millard, C. K. The supposed infectivity of desquamation in Scarlet Fever. Transactions of Epidemiological Society. New Series, Vol. XXI. 1902.

Higgins, T. S. The Bacillus Diphtheriæ in relation to "Return cases" of Scarlet Fever. Public Health, April, 1912.

Arnold, M. B. The period of infectivity in Scarlatina. Public Health, August, 1911.

CHAPTER XIV

STAFF REQUIRED FOR AN ISOLATION HOSPITAL

THE power given to local authorities by § 131, Public Health Act, 1875, to provide hospitals, includes the power to provide medical attendance, nursing and other things necessary for the sick.

The staff required for an isolation hospital must be decided by the local authority themselves in each case, according to the size of the hospital and the number and character of the cases treated in it, together with local and personal considerations which will vary from time to time. The following remarks have reference especially to the structural accommodation which it may be necessary to provide.

Medical Staff. The functions of the medical staff will include not only the treatment of the patients, but also the medical superintendence of the establishment, including such duties as supervision over its sanitary condition, the allotment of wards to different classes of cases and the discipline of the institution ; the arrangements for the removal of patients to hospital and the discharge of convalescents, as well as the consideration of general lines of treatment to be adopted.

These duties may be best discharged by the medical officer of health, if he has time, but they do not fall within his duties as defined by the orders of the late Local Government Board, and if they are placed on him, the remuneration paid to him for them must be separate from his salary as medical officer of health, since the local authority are not entitled to any repayment in respect of it from county funds.

Where the hospital contains some 30—50 beds and is in more or less constant use, the appointment of a resident medical officer may become necessary, especially if the hospital is not convenient of access; but the medical officer of health, if circumstances permit, may still act as visiting or consulting physician and retain a general medical supervision over the working of the hospital.   In such cases the resident medical officer, who may also act as assistant medical officer of health, is generally a junior practitioner, and a lady has sometimes been appointed to the office.   The resident medical officer, if living in the administration block, should have a suite of apartments separate from the nurses' rooms.   If furnished with a laboratory he may usefully undertake bacteriological work for the purposes of the general sanitary administration of the district as well as examinations for the hospital.

In bigger hospitals a larger medical staff will, of course, be required.   In more populous cities, or where the medical officer of health acts for an extensive combination of districts or resides at a distance from the hospital, he will generally be unable to undertake any executive duties in connection with it, but even then it is desirable that he should be in general touch with the hospital administration, and that there should be co-operation between him and the medical superintendent in regard to such matters as the number and nature of cases for which hospital accommodation is likely to be required, the nature of cases sent in under a wrong diagnosis, the occurrence of "return cases," etc.

Where the hospital is of any considerable size, the medical officer in charge will probably be a practitioner of longer standing for whom it may be thought desirable to provide a house at the hospital, though not actually within the same curtilage.

In the earlier history of isolation hospitals, when consent on the part of patients and their friends and medical attendants to removal to hospital was often difficult to obtain, it was not infrequently the practice to allow the patient to continue to be attended in hospital by his own doctor, usually at the patient's own cost, pauper patients being attended by the poor law medical officer.   But at the present time medical practitioners are more often glad to be spared the duty of attending infectious cases, with a view to avoiding risk or alarm to their other patients, and the attendance on the inmates is usually left in the hands of the hospital medical officer.   A consultation with the patient's own doctor may be permitted if desired.

The general and financial control of the hospital should be in the hands of a duly appointed and responsible committee to whom the medical superintendent will report.

Caretakers.   A hospital, however small, if it is to be kept in readiness for the reception of patients at a few hours' notice, requires to be constantly looked after to see that it is kept in a state of proper repair, clean and dry.

Very small hospitals which are often empty may be put in charge of a middle-aged woman, who lives in or near the hospital, to look after it when it is empty, and to undertake cooking, washing, etc. when there are patients in it; matters requiring a man's attention being in the hands of the sanitary inspector or other employé of the local authority.   A frequent arrangement at small hospitals is to appoint a married couple, without children, as caretakers.   The man may have been in one of the public services, or may be employed by the District Council in some other capacity when there are no patients in the hospital.   When the hospital is in use the man acts as porter, messenger, etc., and his wife does the cooking and other household duties, and may even attend on one or two patients if they are not seriously ill, otherwise nurses are engaged as required.   The arrangement has the advantage of being economical, where the hospital is often empty, but its satisfactory working depends upon both of the couple possessing the necessary qualities. To avoid occasions of friction the apartments of the caretakers should be separate from those of the nurses, and the places and duties of each should be clearly defined.

In hospitals above the smallest a matron with proper qualifications should be appointed, and in large hospitals a steward will be needed. The matron is usually given a sitting-room and office and a good-sized bedroom.

Servants. Accommodation should be provided for a sufficient number of servants, as it is undesirable that persons employed at the hospital, especially those whose duties bring them in contact with infection as laundresses, should live outside with their families or in lodgings, and go to and from work. Sleeping accommodation for servants may be provided in dormitories containing several beds.

Nurses. The maintenance of an efficient staff of nurses at a small hospital presents difficulties owing to the varying number of patients, and this is one of the reasons for which such hospitals are unadvisable, if by combination a more workable size can be secured. To keep up a full staff of nurses at a time when there may be few or no patients in hospital is an expense for which there is no return. On the other hand, if nurses are discharged it may be difficult to get them together again when required. The charges made by nursing institutions for nurses for infectious cases are higher than for ordinary cases, and a "scratch team" of nurses is likely to work less well together than a staff who have been instructed in similar methods.

It is desirable that every hospital, however small, which professes to be kept in readiness for patients should have at least one trained nurse permanently engaged, who may act as matron or caretaker, with the aid of a servant, when the hospital is empty, and may perhaps at such times find occupation as a district nurse.

With a view to reducing the cost of upkeep of staff at times when there are few or no patients in hospital, a scheme (appended) has been approved by the Gloucestershire and Worcestershire County Councils and the Town Councils of Bristol, Gloucester, and Worcester, for the interchange of nurses between one hospital and another as the needs of each may require. The nurses whose services are not required at the time by the hospital authority engaging them, may, while still remaining the servants of that authority and receiving from them their usual pay, be lent to other hospitals for a payment of £1. 1s. per week, or £1. 11s. 6d. in the case of small-pox, of which sum the nurse receives one-third. This arrangement it was hoped would be of advantage all round. The hospitals would be able to maintain a smaller permanent staff than would otherwise be necessary, since they would be able to engage the services of additional nurses on occasions of pressure at a cheaper rate than by hiring from a nursing institution, and they would also be relieved of the cost of the keep of unemployed nurses. The nurses on the other hand would receive additional payment for the times when their services were lent to other authorities.

Dr Middleton Martin, County Medical Officer of Health for Gloucestershire, states, however, that the full benefit expected from the scheme has not been realised, partly owing to the general character of the hospitals in the area, partly to the lack of enterprise of the majority of the hospital authorities and their want of appreciation of the economy that could be effected. During the six years that the scheme has been in operation the names of only 23 nurses available for work outside their own hospitals have been sent in; and during the same period there were 109 applications for nurses, but only 29 could be supplied. On one occasion, however, during an outbreak of small-pox, the prompt loan of two nurses by one hospital was greatly appreciated. Apparently few hospitals in the area keep a sufficient staff of nurses to be able to spare any, even during slack times.

NURSES EXCHANGE FOR ISOLATION HOSPITALS IN THE ADMINISTRATIVE COUNTIES OF GLOUCESTERSHIRE AND WORCESTERSHIRE AND THE CITIES OF BRISTOL, GLOUCESTER AND WORCESTER.

SCHEME prepared by the county medical officers for Gloucestershire and Worcestershire, as amended and approved by committee appointed at conference held at Gloucester on 12th May, 1906, to frame in detail a scheme for loan of nurses between isolation hospitals, and as approved at a conference of Gloucestershire and Worcestershire hospital authorities held on the 13th October, 1906.

Adopted by the Gloucestershire County Council on the 22nd day of October, 1906, and the Worcestershire County Council on the 10th day of December, 1906.

1. Registers of nurses available for work to be kept—one for the county of Gloucester and the cities associated with it, and one for the county of Worcester and the city of Worcester.

2. The county councils of such administrative counties to be asked to keep such registers, and to act as centres of communication.

3. Any isolation hospital authority participating in the scheme who
    (1) Have nurses available—(the " Lending Hospital ") ;
    (2) Require nurses   —(the " Borrowing Hospital "),
to communicate with the centre for their area, giving such particulars as may be arranged.

4. Each centre to satisfy the needs of its area as far as it is able. If at any time either centre should not have a nurse available, it shall put the borrowing hospital in communication with the other centre.

5. When requested, the registration centre to put the borrowing hospital authority into communication with a lending hospital authority, but the arrangement for the actual transfer of the nurses, and the payment of the fees according to the scale, to be made directly by the hospital committees concerned.

6. The fees payable in respect of such services by the borrowing to the lending hospital shall be :—
    (1) For nursing small-pox—
        1½ guineas per week (trained nurse).
        1 guinea per week (probationer of not less than one year's service).
    (2) Other diseases than small-pox—
        1 guinea per week (trained nurse).
        15s. per week (probationer of not less than one year's service).
    Travelling expenses (including third-class railway fare) each way will be paid by the borrowing hospital.

7. The term " nurse " where hereafter used in this scheme shall include a probationer.

8. One-third of the fee received by the lending authority, together with travelling expenses, shall be paid to the nurse in addition to her salary, to compensate her for moving.

9. A borrowed nurse may be recalled or returned on 24 hours' notice being given. Any hospital giving up a nurse to have the first claim on any other available nurse at either of the centres.

10. A borrowed nurse, for the time of borrowing, to be subject to the rules of the borrowing hospital, and to undertake either day or night work, as may be required, and in cases of emergency, if she expresses her willingness to do so, she may undertake both day and night work.

11. If a borrowed nurse considers she has reason to complain of the treatment she receives, or of the rules under which she is compelled to act, at the hospital of the borrowing authority, she shall be at liberty to submit a written complaint to the borrowing authority, through the officer in charge of the hospital of such authority, and in such case shall send a copy of such complaint

to the lending authority, and, in the event of the borrowing authority failing to deal promptly with such complaint to the satisfaction of the lending authority, such authority shall be entitled to withdraw their nurse on giving 24 hours' notice to the borrowing authority.

12. The committee of the borrowing hospital shall arrange for the disinfection of the borrowed nurse's clothing, and the matron of the borrowing hospital shall inform the matron of the lending hospital as to the particular disease the borrowed nurse has been last attending, in order that the medical officer of the lending hospital may be satisfied that the nurse in question cannot convey infection from the borrowing to the lending hospital.

13. Any hospital authority, whose hospital is placed outside the counties of Gloucester and Worcester, but who provides accommodation for districts inside either of those counties, may participate in this scheme on the conditions named above, and communications shall be addressed to the centre in which the district served by such hospital is situated.

Comfortable quarters should be provided, as the nurses at an isolation hospital are much debarred from outside society by the nature of their calling and the precautions required against spreading infection. At temporary hospitals difficulty has sometimes been experienced in obtaining nurses from nursing institutions on account of the unsatisfactory accommodation provided for them. A separate bedroom should, if possible, be provided for each nurse, and in reckoning the number to be provided it may be assumed that each ward-block may require at least one day nurse and one night nurse, who should have separate bedrooms. Nurses should not be allowed to sleep in the ward-blocks or duty rooms. A greater number of nurses, who will probably be classified in grades, will be required in large wards.

The modern methods of aseptic nursing described in the chapter on Bed Isolation (Chapter XII) will necessitate a larger proportion of nurses, who will need to be highly-trained.

Even at large fever hospitals, such as those of the Metropolitan Asylums Board, it has not always been found easy to maintain a staff of nurses of satisfactory qualifications, and a new scheme for the nursing staff was adopted by that Board in 1910.

An arrangement, such as has sometimes existed, by which the nurses are boarded by contract with the matron is an undesirable one.

At large hospitals arrangements are made for receiving probationers for training.

At small-pox hospitals the nurses, and indeed all the staff, should be protected by recent and efficient re-vaccination.

BIBLIOGRAPHY

Nightingale, Florence. Notes on Hospitals. 1863.
Thorne. Hospital Report. 1882.
Chalmers, Dr (M.O.H. Glasgow). Memorandum on Hospitals. 1910.
Barwise, Dr S. Report on the Isolation Hospitals of Derbyshire. 1906.
Metropolitan Asylums Board, Annual Report. 1910.
Gordon, A. Knyvett. Some practical points in the management of an Isolation Hospital. Public Health, March, 1905.

CHAPTER XV

INFECTIOUS DISEASE AND THE POOR LAW

It has been already mentioned in Chapter I that the hospital treatment of infectious diseases was first taken up by official bodies as a measure of poor relief, wards for such diseases being provided at the workhouse infirmaries by the board of guardians. The relation between poverty and infectious diseases is twofold; on the one hand poverty leads to insufficient nutrition, overcrowding and uncleanly surroundings, and thus predisposes to infectious diseases; on the other hand the occurrence of infectious disease, especially in the breadwinner of the household, may itself be the cause of destitution requiring relief. The latter was probably the case in former years to a greater extent than now; for in the period between the passing of the Public Health Acts of 1848 and 1872 there were frequent epidemics of typhus, relapsing fever, cholera and small-pox—diseases liable to attack adults—but since 1872 the age-incidence of infectious diseases has shifted, and the prevalent diseases now are scarlet fever, diphtheria, measles and whooping-cough, diseases chiefly of childhood, and therefore most frequent in the section of the population having the largest proportion of children, that is to say, generally the artizan and labourer class. Better wages have rendered this class less dependent on the Poor Law; for these reasons hospitals for infectious diseases are now required not so much as a means for relieving destitution as for controlling the spread of infectious disease.

The duties of boards of guardians in relation to infectious disease are thus set forth by the late Local Government Board:

> "Where a person suffering from illness, including infectious disease, is destitute, it is the duty of the Guardians, or in the interval between their meetings, of the relieving officer, to give such relief as the case may require, and if necessary to arrange for the admission of the patient to a hospital. Where however such removal is only required for purposes of isolation and the person to be removed is not destitute, the Guardians have no duty, and the necessary provision should be made by the Sanitary Authority. The test of the Guardians' duty in the matter is the destitution of the patient, and this will not necessarily depend upon his being in the actual receipt of relief, but may consist in his being unable to obtain at his own cost the requisite medical attendance, nursing and accommodation[1]."

This ruling, viz. that the relief of destitution was a matter for the guardians, and the isolation of the patient with a view to prevent the spread of disease a matter for the sanitary authority[2], was not in all cases carried out without difficulty. Border cases were often met with in which the two duties were not easily separable; the number of cases requiring treatment in the workhouse fever hospitals, for the reasons already mentioned, proved to be more limited than had been anticipated; and it seemed anomalous that there should be no place to which patients whose

---

[1] The converse of this statement, viz. that sanitary authorities are concerned only with proper isolation and have no duties where admission to a hospital is required only for the purpose of treatment, does not hold good. The powers of local authorities under § 131, Public Health Act, 1875, do not relate only to hospitals for infectious diseases; and they may, and some do, admit into their isolation hospitals diseases such as puerperal fever, erysipelas, ophthalmia of newborn infants, measles and whooping-cough, with a view to save the life and prevent the disablement of the patient, rather than to prevent the spread of the disease to others.

[2] § 22, Poor Law Amendment Act, 1867, gives power to the guardians to detain in the workhouse any poor persons suffering from an infectious or contagious disease who is not in a proper state to leave the workhouse without danger to himself or others.

Under § 84, Public Health Act, 1875, the keeper of a common lodging house, when a person in such house is ill of fever or any infectious disease, is required to give notice thereof not only to the medical officer of health of the local authority, but also to the poor law relieving officer of the union or parish in which the common lodging house is situated.

isolation was urgently required could be taken, while at the same time what was regarded as a good hospital, built perhaps under pressure from the central authority, was standing empty, or that while there was such a hospital the sanitary authority should be put to the expense of providing another.

The eventual solution of the difficulty was found in opposite directions in London and in the provinces. In London the Metropolitan Asylums Board, in its origin a Poor Law body, became eventually the isolation hospital authority for the whole population of London, pauper and non-pauper, as will be narrated in the next chapter.

Outside London the provision of isolation hospital accommodation is now generally recognised to be the function of the sanitary authority, acting alone or in combination with other authorities, or of the County Council, under the Isolation Hospital Acts, and the guardians commonly make an arrangement with them for the reception into the hospital, on settled terms, of infectious cases among paupers.

It is very desirable that such an agreement should be entered into beforehand in all cases, in order to avoid delay and disputes, unless the sanitary authority are willing to take all cases without payment. It might seem at first sight immaterial, if the expenses are to be paid out of the rates in any case, whether they were paid by one body or another, and if the districts of the two were coextensive this might be so; but in practice owing to the overlapping of districts and the unequal incidence of rating, disputes are apt to arise in the absence of an agreement. For instance, in the agricultural counties a poor law union often consists of a market town which forms an urban district and a number of surrounding parishes forming a rural district. The urban district council has provided an isolation hospital, but the rural district council has not done so. An emergency occurs, *e.g.* a casual at the workhouse or on the road is discovered to have small-pox, and a hurried application is made to the urban district council to have him admitted to the hospital. To avoid delay no formalities are insisted on and the man is admitted. When the account is sent in the guardians, among whom the representatives of the rural parishes are in a majority, refuse to pay, and the terms of § 132, Public Health Act, 1875, as guardians have sometimes been advised[1], do not enable the urban council to recover the cost from them in the absence of a formal agreement. The guardians thus escape paying on this occasion, but the urban district council will naturally not be willing to admit similar cases another time[2].

Casual paupers and small-pox. Frequent instances have occurred in which infectious diseases, especially small-pox, have been introduced into a district by persons of vagrant habits who sleep in casual wards, night refuges and common lodging houses, where they are liable to come into contact with a number of other persons of similar habits. A person suffering from small-pox in an early stage, before the nature of the disease has been detected, or a mild and unrecognised case, may thus impart infection to a number of other persons; and these during the 12 to 14 days over which the incubation period of the disease extends, may wander about the country and eventually start the infection in like manner in other districts. This is, indeed, one of the ways in which outbreaks of small-pox most often arise. The Local Government Board in 1893 issued the following letter to boards of guardians advising them what precautions should be taken in order to guard against this danger.

LOCAL GOVERNMENT BOARD, WHITEHALL, S.W.,
13th February 1893.

SIR,

I am directed by the Local Government Board to state that they have had recently brought under their attention a number of instances in which casual paupers who have been admitted to the casual wards have been found to be suffering from small-pox, and on several occasions it has appeared that the persons so affected had, on the night immediately preceding their application for admission to the casual wards, slept in other casual wards.

There is no doubt that there is considerable risk of small-pox being spread

---

[1] But see the case of The Queen *v.* Mayor, etc., of Rawtenstall mentioned on p. 147, Chap. XI. In that case however an agreement had been made between the guardians and the corporation for the reception into the latter's hospital of pauper patients on payment by the guardians, though the corporation afterwards repudiated it.

[2] A similar repudiation has sometimes happened when one district council has in an emergency admitted into its hospital cases from the district of another district council without requiring from the latter a previous undertaking to pay.

by means of casual paupers, and the Board trust that the guardians and their officers will take such measures as will tend as far as possible to diminish this danger.

The regulations of the Board relative to the relief of casual paupers, which were issued on the 18th December 1882, by Article 13 provide that in the event of any casual pauper being ill the master of the workhouse or the superintendent of the casual wards shall, as soon as practicable, obtain the attendance of the medical officer, who shall give directions as to the treatment of such pauper. The Board consider it a matter of great importance that the attention of the medical officer should be at once called to any casual pauper who may complain of illness, or who, in the absence of complaint, may present any suspicious symptoms, and they request that the guardians will be so good as to give such instructions to the master of the workhouse or superintendent of the casual wards as will ensure that this shall be done, and that the greatest vigilance may be exercised to check the discharge of persons who are likely to be suffering from small-pox, or, being convalescent, may still be a source of danger to others.

The regulations of the Board contemplate that under ordinary circumstances a casual pauper when ill shall be removed to the workhouse ; but the guardians will realise that, as a general rule, patients suffering from small-pox cannot be retained on the workhouse premises without very serious risk of the spread of the disease.

The Sanitary Authorities are expressly empowered by section 131 of the Public Health Act to provide hospital accommodation for the isolation of persons suffering from dangerous infectious disease, and when the Sanitary Authority have provided a hospital suitable for the reception of small-pox cases the Board consider that the guardians should, if possible, arrange beforehand with the Sanitary Authority for the reception into such hospital, when necessary, of any persons suffering from small-pox for whom relief is required.

The Board are advised that, as a general rule, only circumstances of grave urgency justify the admission or retention of a small-pox case in a workhouse. The guardians, when there is no hospital already provided by the Sanitary Authority affording suitable accommodation, should immediately consider, in concert with the Medical Officer of Health, what other provision for the due isolation of patients is practicable.

The Board must, at the same time, observe that when a case of small-pox occurs, whether in the casual wards or in the workhouse, and indeed in times of small-pox prevalence generally, it is, in the opinion of the Board, of the greatest importance that measures should at once be taken to secure, as far as practicable, vaccination or re-vaccination of the other inmates, so far as the medical officer may consider needful. Care should especially be taken that the nurses and other persons employed to attend upon the patients or brought into personal contact with them should be such as have, within a sufficiently recent period, been either successfully re-vaccinated or had small-pox ; or, when there is a difficulty in securing this, that such persons should at once be re-vaccinated as a protection against the disease.

The Board request that whenever there is an occurrence of small-pox or any other dangerous infectious disease in a workhouse, including any case occurring in the casual wards, the fact may be immediately reported to them by the medical officer, with a statement showing for each case the date of attack and source of infection, so far as may be known. The medical officer should also state what provision has been made for preventing the spread of the disease among the inmates, and for the isolation and nursing of the patients, and whether he is satisfied of the sufficiency of such provision. In the case of small-pox occurring the medical officer should fully inform the Board of such measures as may be taken in regard to vaccination and re-vaccination.

I am, Sir,

Your obedient Servant,

HUGH OWEN,

Secretary.

The Clerk to the Guardians.

Workhouse Infectious Hospitals as Isolation Hospitals. In view of the little use often made of the fever hospital erected in connection with the workhouse, while at the same time there might be much need for an isolation hospital for the general use of the district, the workhouse infectious hospital building has in some cases, where it was suitable for the purpose, been leased by the guardians to the sanitary authority with the consent of the Local Government Board. Three such instances are mentioned in Sir R. Thorne's Report, viz. the hospitals in connection with the workhouses at Goole, Settle, and Warwick, but in all these cases the lease has now lapsed, the building being required for workhouse purposes, and a new isolation hospital has been built for the general use of the district. At Bicester, however, the workhouse fever building continues to be used as an isolation hospital for the urban and rural districts[1].

The Bicester, Goole and Settle hospitals are all nearly on the same plan, which may have been a model one in use under the Poor Law Board. The description of the Goole hospital will illustrate their general arrangement.

> The Goole workhouse infectious hospital is a substantial brick building of two storeys, situated behind the other workhouse buildings, and approached by a roadway through the workhouse curtilage by the side of the other buildings. It stands in a garden which was separated from the rest of the workhouse grounds by a high brick wall, built when the hospital was leased to the Local Board.

[1] At Ticehurst a building erected originally as the workhouse fever block has been transferred from the guardians to the rural district council, and adapted for use as the isolation hospital for the district. It is near the workhouse, but on a detached site.

At the back it is very near the boundary of the site. On the ground floor in the centre of the building there is a kitchen and a nurse's day room ; on either side of these is an entrance lobby, with a stone staircase leading to the upper floor; out of this lobby leads a ward 24 × 20 ft. and 12 ft. high; and beyond this ward at either end of the building is another smaller ward 18 × 20 ft. with a separate entrance from the open air. The same arrangement of wards is repeated on the upper floor. There are thus 8 wards, supposed to hold 20 or 24 beds, and affording accommodation for the simultaneous treatment of two diseases in both sexes. The administration accommodation however, which was designed for a hospital to be worked from the workhouse, was quite inadequate to the requirements of a hospital to be administered independently ; thus there was originally no place for the storage of food and a larder had to be built in a somewhat inconvenient position. The position of the wards, especially the end wards on the upper floor, was inconvenient for nursing ; the arrangement of the w.c.s was defective and the position of the bath rooms, on the upper floor, inconvenient. The water supply was pumped from a well on the workhouse premises. The close association of the building with the workhouse had been found to militate against its use.

In cases where the transference of a workhouse hospital to the sanitary authority needed the consent of the Local Government Board, the Board required as conditions of their approval that the building could be spared for workhouse use ; that it was capable of complete severance from the workhouse, and was, or would be, provided with separate means of administration, and a separate entrance from the public road. It must also be so situated with respect to the workhouse that risk of infection to the latter need not be apprehended ; every infected building must be at least 40 feet from the boundary and cases of small-pox must not be received. The building must be substantially constructed and in good sanitary condition, and the grounds must be fenced in accordance with usual requirements. There must be accommodation for a sufficient staff, and suitable outbuildings, drainage and water supply independent of the workhouse ; except in very small districts there should be facilities for the reception at one time of two different infectious diseases in both sexes. But it is only in comparatively few instances that workhouse infectious wards have been found sufficiently detached from other workhouse buildings, and capable of separate administration, so as to permit of their use as isolation hospitals, and, even then, their close association with the workhouse is a disadvantage.

Sir R. Thorne speaks of the possibility that the admission

of paupers, and especially of indoor paupers in workhouse uniform, into an isolation hospital might deter the non-pauper classes from seeking admission, and he states that on this ground some hospital authorities made it a rule to refuse admission to any person in receipt of relief from the guardians. He advises that pauper patients should be provided with suits belonging to the hospital and should not be attended by the workhouse staff. We have not heard of difficulty on this score being experienced in recent years. It is not improbable that some sweeping changes may occur in the near future in Poor Law Administration and presumably in its relation to infectious disease, but it is not possible at the present time to predict what the results of these changes will be.

BIBLIOGRAPHY

Reports of the Local Government Board, passim.
Report of the Hospital Commission. 1882.
Copnall. Law of Infectious Diseases and Hospitals. 1899.
Thorne. Hospital Report. 1882.
Low, J. Spencer. Report to the Local Government Board on the Sanitary Circumstances and Administration of the Hawarden Rural District. 1907.
Armstrong, H. E. Small-pox and Vagrancy. 1893-4.

CHAPTER XVI

HOSPITAL SYSTEM OF THE METROPOLITAN ASYLUMS BOARD

In London, hospital provision for infectious diseases has followed different lines from those in the rest of the kingdom.

Although by § 37 of the Sanitary Act, 1866, sanitary authorities in London were given power to provide hospitals and this power is continued by § 75, Public Health (London) Act, 1891, very few of these authorities have exercised this power; and the function of providing hospital accommodation for persons suffering from infectious diseases has passed by degrees into the hands of the Metropolitan Asylums Board, which is in its origin and relations a body for the relief of the poor.

The circumstances which gave rise to the formation of the Metropolitan Asylums Board have been already mentioned in

Chapter I. Prior to its formation, the only places in London for the reception of persons suffering from infectious diseases were:

1st. The Highgate Small-Pox Hospital and the London Fever Hospital at Islington. These were charitable foundations, but a certain payment was required from patients: some cases also were sent in by boards of guardians on payment.

2nd. Fever cases admitted into the general hospitals.

3rd. The workhouse infirmaries, some of which had fever wards. These belonged to the boards of guardians of 31 parishes or unions, and were maintained out of the rates of the parishes or unions which they served, the cost falling heaviest on the poorest parishes. The cases in them "were nursed and cared for by other paupers. These pauper nurses were as a rule feeble old men and women, who knew nothing about nursing, whose previous careers had in many instances been vicious, whose love of drink often led them to beg or buy from or rob the sick of the stimulants provided for them, and whose treatment of the poor was, generally speaking, not characterised either by judgment or kindness."

On May 15, 1867, the Poor Law Board, under the powers of the Metropolitan Poor Law Act, 1867, by an Order constituted a Board of Managers of the Metropolitan Asylum District, to make provision "for the reception and relief of the classes of poor persons chargeable to some Union or Parish in the said district who may be infected with or suffering from fever, or the disease of small-pox, or may be insane."

The Board of Managers consisted partly of representatives of the several boards of guardians, partly of members nominated by the Poor Law Board, afterwards the Local Government Board and now the Ministry of Health. It was prescribed in 1875 that " The insane paupers to be taken into the asylum shall be such harmless persons of the chronic or imbecile class as could be lawfully detained in the workhouse. No dangerous or curable persons such as would under the statutes in that behalf require to be sent to a lunatic asylum shall be admitted." In the same year the Managers were authorised to provide a ship for training boys for the sea service; and in 1897 they were empowered to provide accommodation for certain special classes of children chargeable to the guardians, viz. :

(*a*)   Children suffering from ophthalmia or other contagious disease of the eye.

(*b*)   Children suffering from contagious disease of the skin or scalp.

(*c*)   Children requiring either special treatment during convalescence or the benefit of seaside air.

(*d*)   Children who by reason of defect of intellect or physical infirmity cannot properly be trained in association with children in ordinary schools.

(*e*)   Children who are ordered by two justices or a magistrate to be taken, under the Industrial Schools Act, 1866, to a workhouse or an asylum of the district.

On 10th Nov., 1911, the Local Government Board issued an Order constituting the Metropolitan Asylums Board the authority for the relief of the casual poor of the Metropolis. From 1st April, 1912, the control of 24 casual wards previously administered by the separate boards of guardians has been centralised under the Asylums Board.

The Managers had been empowered in 1879 to undertake the removal of patients from their homes to the hospitals. This had previously been in the hands of the guardians, and was often effected with unsuitable vehicles and subject to frequent irregularities.

The present work of the Metropolitan Asylums Board falls therefore under six heads ; viz.:

1.   Hospitals for infectious diseases.
2.   Ambulance service.
3.   Imbecile asylums.
4.   Training ship.
5.   Special classes of children.
6.   Casual paupers.

Of these, the four latter are concerned solely with paupers, and need not be further referred to.

The hospitals for infectious diseases were also at first limited to pauper cases, admittance being by a relieving officer's order, accompanied by a certificate from the district medical officer under the Poor Law. The accommodation at first provided was therefore on a scale to suffice for paupers only. Sites were obtained at Homerton, Stockwell and Hampstead, and plans were prepared for a permanent fever hospital and small-pox hospital on each site. Before, however, the permanent hospitals were completed the Managers were compelled to erect temporary buildings to meet an outbreak of relapsing fever in 1869, and subsequently to cope with the formidable epidemic of small-pox in 1870—71. Additional sites at Deptford and Fulham were acquired during the small-pox epidemic of 1876—8, and rapidly covered with hospital buildings, and other sites since then have been acquired and hospitals built from time to time.

Between 1871 and 1885—as indeed before 1871—small-pox was continually more or less prevalent in London, recurring as an epidemic every third or fourth year. The story of how the small-pox hospitals were found to act as centres for the dissemination of the disease around them: how the subject was inquired into by a Royal Commission in 1882: how from 1886 all small-pox cases were removed to hospitals out of London: and how the disease thereupon practically ceased to be endemic in London has been told in Chapter IX.

The evidence given before the Royal Commission showed that a very large proportion of the cases received into the Managers' Hospitals were not strictly paupers, and only sought admission because they could not be efficiently nursed or safely isolated at their own homes ; but by their admission they became paupers, entailing loss of civil privileges, such as the vote.

The Royal Commission recommended that instead of the isolation of non-pauper cases of infectious disease being left to the sanitary authorities (then vestries and district boards some 39 in number) there should be a single hospital authority for the whole of London[1], and that this should be in its general aspect not a pauper but a sanitary authority, the guardians and sanitary authorities being both represented in its composition. They also recommended :

That the provision of hospital accommodation for infectious

[1] The London County Council was not then in existence.

disease should be entirely disconnected from the poor law, and be treated as part of the sanitary arrangements of London :

That cases of infectious disease should be notified to the medical officer of health of the district in which the patient resides :

That the hospitals hitherto used for small-pox should in the main become fever hospitals, and small-pox should be treated in hospitals established in isolated situations on the banks of the Thames or in floating hospitals on the river itself : and

That convalescent hospitals for infectious cases should be established at some distance in the country.

In 1883 an Act was passed removing the civil disabilities attaching to admission into the Managers' Hospitals. The regulation requiring that every patient should be admitted on a relieving officer's order was so far relaxed as to allow admission on the receipt of information from any poor law official on condition that the prescribed "admission order" was subsequently sent. In 1887 the certificate of any registered medical practitioner was accepted in place of that of the poor law medical officer.

In 1889 the Asylums Board were empowered by Act of Parliament, subject to the regulations of the Local Government Board, to admit into their hospitals any person who is reasonably believed to be suffering from fever, small-pox or diphtheria, but the guardians still retained the power to recover the cost of their maintenance from non-pauper patients or their legally liable relatives.

By § 80, Public Health (London) Act, 1891, it was enacted that the expenses incurred by the Managers for the maintenance of any person not a pauper, should be paid by the board of guardians of the poor law union from which he is received, but these expenses shall be repaid to the guardians out of the metropolitan common poor fund. The admission of a person suffering from an infectious disease into any hospital provided by the Managers and his maintenance therein are not to be considered parochial relief, alms, or charitable allowance, and are not to entail deprivation of any right or privilege or render him subject to any disability or disqualification. Thus hospital accommodation is now available free of cost for every inhabitant of London suffering from infectious disease, and its use involves no pauperisation, although it is provided and paid for through poor law channels.

The effect of this removal of restrictions is shown in the following table taken from the evidence of Mr T. Duncombe Mann, clerk to the Board, before the Royal Commission on the Poor Laws in 1906.

Groups of Years	Average annual number of admissions to Board's Hospitals				Average annual mortality in London per 1000 estimated population			
	Scarlet fever	Typhus	Enteric	Diphtheria	Scarlet fever	Typhus	Enteric	Diphtheria
I. 1871–1878. (Admissions confined to pauper class)	502	202	317	—	0·56	0·60	0·25	—
II. 1879–1886. (Regulations as to admissions slightly relaxed)	1705	72	387	—	0·48	0·01	0·21	—
III. 1887–1891. (Regulations as to admissions further relaxed)	5325	19	487	992	0·24	0·00	0·15	0·32
IV. 1892–1899. (All restrictive regulations removed, and use of hospitals free)	13,377	7	729	4697	0·21	0·00	0·14	0·54
V. 1900–1905	13,040	7	1097	5970	0·10	0·00	0·155	0·23

The proportion of admissions to hospital to the total number of legally admissible cases increased from 33·6 per cent. in 1890, the year when notification of infectious diseases first came into force, to 84·6 per cent. in 1905, near which point it has since remained. In 1911 the proportion was 84·3 for all legally admissible cases, viz. 89·2 per cent. of scarlet fever cases notified, 85·0 per cent. of diphtheria, 50·6 per cent. of enteric fever, and 98·6 per cent. of small-pox.

In the earlier years of the Board's existence its energies had especially to be devoted to coping with epidemics of small-pox. Typhus fever was also frequent at that time, but is now rare in London. Relapsing fever has not recurred since the outbreak in 1869. Scarlet fever cases are by far the most numerous of those admitted. Enteric fever is a much smaller cause of mortality in London at the present time than in past years, but the proportion of cases which are admitted to the Asylums Board's hospitals has increased.

Diphtheria cases were not admitted into the Asylums Board's hospitals before 1888, owing to a doubt as to whether this disease came within the term "fever," but its admission was expressly authorised by the Act of 1889. Measles and whooping-cough were made admissible in 1910. A considerable number of cases of other diseases, amounting in 1911 to 10·6 per cent. of the whole, are also sent in on erroneous diagnoses, notwithstanding that a medical certificate is required as a condition of admission in every case.

It has often been suggested that the hospitals of the Metropolitan Asylums Board, when not in use for fever or small-pox, should be utilised for cases of tuberculosis. The arrangements authorised by § 16, National Insurance Act, 1911, for administering sanatorium benefit can only be made with local authorities other than Poor Law authorities ; but § 39 of the National Insurance Act, 1913, renders it lawful for the Metropolitan Asylums Board to enter into agreement with any county council or county borough council for the reception of *insured* persons and their dependents suffering from tuberculosis.

The great increase in the number of patients admitted to the Metropolitan Asylums Board's hospitals—due partly to a greater number of diseases being admissible, but to a still greater extent to their being made available for larger and larger sections of the community, and to a more general readiness to make use of them—has necessitated the provision of a large amount of accommodation beyond what was at first anticipated as necessary. New hospitals have been established from time to time, and existing hospitals have been extended. At the end of 1911 the Managers possessed 14 hospitals for infectious diseases, of which 11, with 6528 beds, were for fevers and diphtheria; eight, with 4259 beds, being town hospitals, and two, with 2269 beds, being convalescent hospitals situated several miles outside London. For small-pox there are three hospitals, with an aggregate of 2040 beds, situated near Dartford, in Kent, and accessible from the river Thames.

The earlier hospital buildings erected by the Managers, and some of the later ones, were wooden structures, this method of construction being adopted to save time, as the hospitals were hurriedly provided under the pressure of epidemics. But the disadvantages of temporary buildings having been experienced— they were inadequate, out-of-date, dangerous in respect of fire risk, and expensive to maintain—the later hospitals have been permanent buildings of brick, mostly of two storeys.

At the time of the small-pox epidemic of 1871 the Managers purchased a hospital ship, the "Dreadnought," moored in the Thames off Greenwich, as a convalescent hospital for small-pox patients : this was afterwards replaced by two ships, the "Atlas" and "Endymion." Later on, about 1884, these vessels were moved down the Thames to Long Reach, near Dartford, about 17 miles from London, and moored near an uninhabited part of the Kentish shore, administrative buildings for use in connection with them being built on shore. At the same time the Managers purchased the "Castalia," a twin-ship specially designed for the channel traffic between Dover and Calais, but which had proved unsuitable for that purpose, and fitted her up as a hospital. The engines and paddle wheels were removed, and the interval between the two hulls was decked over, forming an upper and a lower hospital. The lower deck was divided into five wards, and on the upper platform were constructed five wards, placed *en échelon* with reception room, isolation wards, bathrooms, etc. The vessel accommodated altogether 150 patients. It was warmed by steam pipes from an adjoining vessel, which was used also for administration purposes.

For the transport of small-pox patients four ambulance steamboats have been provided. There are also three wharves for their embarkation situated on the banks of the Thames at convenient places. The patients, who are brought by road ambulances, are examined on their arrival at the wharf by a medical officer, who confirms the diagnosis or otherwise, and decides whether the patient is in a condition to bear the voyage.   If not, or if, as sometimes happens, traffic on the river is suspended by a fog, there are small wards on the wharf into which the patient may be put temporarily.   There are also observation wards for the isolation of doubtful cases.

The hospital ships were however disused in 1904, as certain drawbacks were found to attach to them, especially the liability to injury by passing vessels during a fog, and danger of fire; hospitals on shore in the same neighbourhood have therefore been substituted for them.   The river ambulance service is still continued for the transport of small-pox cases to a wharf where they are disembarked for the land hospitals.

For the transport of fever patients land ambulances are used, and motor vehicles are now being substituted for those which are horse-drawn.   There are six ambulance stations situated in different parts of London.   The Board also provide separate ambulances for the removal of accident and other surgical cases, and of mental and non-infectious medical cases, to general hospitals and elsewhere.

Since 1889 arrangements have been in force for clinical teaching on infectious fevers at the hospitals of the Metropolitan Asylums Board.

The Board publish every year a report which is a mine of statistics relating to infectious diseases, and has a valuable Medical Supplement, containing articles by members of the medical staff of the hospitals.   These reports have been largely quoted from in this book, and the author desires here to express his acknowledgments.

BIBLIOGRAPHY

Report of the Royal Commission on Small-Pox and Fever Hospitals.   1882.
The Metropolitan Asylums Board of London and its Work.   Issued by the
    Board.   1900.
Evidence of Mr T. Duncombe Mann before the Royal Commission on the
    Poor Laws and relief of Distress.   1906.
Annual Report of the Metropolitan Asylums Board for 1911.

CHAPTER XVII

COST OF ISOLATION HOSPITALS

Capital cost. Various circumstances combine to render an isolation hospital a comparatively costly building to erect in proportion to the number of inmates.

Sites are difficult to obtain, as there is often unwillingness to sell land for the purpose of a hospital for infectious disease; in order to obtain one the local authority may have to give a high price per acre, and also to purchase more land than they require or land not very suitable for their purpose. The hospital may have to be placed in a position where no public water service or sewers are at hand, and expense has to be incurred in providing a water supply from a well or spring, and in the disposal of sewage. If the site is remote, the expense of carting materials and procuring labour will be increased, and road making may be needed. As compared with other public institutions such as a workhouse or a lunatic asylum, an isolation hospital is usually on a smaller scale, and therefore the cost of these accessories has to be spread over fewer beds. The inmates, being persons seriously ill, require a comparatively large staff to attend to them, and for this staff accommodation must be provided on the premises. The need for classification of patients involves the provision of small wards, which cost more in proportion than large ones.

For similar reasons the cost per bed of very small hospitals is high as compared with that of larger hospitals, and hence the establishment of very small hospitals is undesirable, where by a combination of districts a single larger hospital would serve. The cost per bed may indeed be diminished by making the wards larger, so that the cost of the other parts of the hospital may be shared by a larger number of beds; but the total cost of the hospital is thereby increased, and without advantage if a smaller number would suffice. From the ratepayer's point of view it is the total cost of the hospital to the district that matters, rather than the cost per bed ; while the sanitary administrator desires to have not so much a large number of beds to meet the contingency of an extensive epidemic as a number sufficient for the ordinary needs of the district, and so arranged in wards as to be useful under the varying circumstances likely to arise.

Assuming that the hospital authority possess a suitable site, with facilities for obtaining a water service and for drainage, the cost of erecting a permanent hospital of medium size, say 20 to 30 beds in two or three ward-blocks, in accordance with the principles set out in the Local Government Board's Memorandum, may be estimated at somewhere about £400 per bed, exclusive of site, varying from £350 to £500, according to circumstances, such as the size of the hospital, the facilities afforded by the site, the style of the buildings and the local prices of labour and materials. Where circumstances are favourable and strict economy is exercised it may be sometimes as low as £300 per bed or even lower, but on the other hand £500 per bed has often been much exceeded, usually through difficulties connected with the site.

Generally speaking, an economical construction of permanent hospitals will be most likely to be secured by following as nearly as possible the lines of the plans in the Local Government Board's Memorandum; any deviation from them, except in the direction of larger wards, usually involving an increased cost per bed. Some saving may perhaps be effected by the use of materials such as concrete, "Frazzi," etc., instead of brick or stone for hospital walls. At Acton a ward-block, built of concrete blocks, cost 4·66d. per cubic foot, as against 6·9d. for brick pavilions[1].

Temporary hospitals, constructed of a wooden frame covered with weather boarding, corrugated iron or other materials may be erected, or bought ready-made, for less than it costs to erect a building of brick or stone, but have serious drawbacks, as already mentioned in Chapter VIII. The ready-made hospitals on the market are commonly deficient in cubic space and administrative accommodation, and the maker's price, it must be remembered,

---

[1] See Memorandum on Sanatoria, appended to Chapter XVIII.

includes only the bare building, exclusive of site, foundations, drainage, water supply, furniture and other requisites, which may cost more than or even twice as much as the building itself.

Sometimes, however, it is possible to buy in the open market a small estate containing an existing dwelling house suitable to serve as an administration block, with land on which temporary ward-blocks can be erected, and in this way a cheap and fairly efficient hospital may be secured, especially if the wards are plastered internally instead of being lined with match-boarding.

Cost of Furnishing. The cost of furnishing hospitals varies greatly in different cases, partly with the size of the hospital, partly according to what is included under the heading of furniture, partly with the views and tendencies of the local authority. In 34 hospitals known to have been completed and furnished, the cost of furniture was on the average £31 per bed, but it ranged from £11 per bed in one case to £62 in another; the latter, however, and several others in which the cost per bed was high, were small hospitals in which the cost of furnishing the administration block (included in the total cost) was shared by very few beds. In nine the cost was below £20 per bed, and in 21 below £30, while in only 11 did it exceed £35. Under ordinary circumstances it should not exceed £35 per bed[1].

The furniture at an isolation hospital should be strong, durable and easily kept clean; but unnecessary articles should be avoided, especially in the wards, and anything like extravagance or display should be eschewed.

Cost of maintenance of isolation hospitals.

Accounts. It is very desirable, as the committee of King Edward's Hospital Fund have often urged, that the accounts of hospitals should be kept on a uniform plan, so that the expenditure of one hospital on each item may be comparable with that of another. Such a comparison has shown the way to effect important savings in the expenditure of the large London general hospitals. There are difficulties in instituting an exact comparison in the case of isolation hospitals, owing to their

[1] It is to be remembered that these estimates were made in 1913, that is, before the war, and therefore before the great rise in prices of material and labour had taken place. It may be some time before pre-war prices are restored.

variation in size and equipment, and in the number of inmates at different times ; indeed there may be periods when they are empty.

Although the accounts of isolation hospitals are subject to audit by the District Auditor, with a view to disallowing any illegal expenditure, the Local Government Board have no power to order that they shall be kept on a uniform plan, except so far as may be necessary in the case of a joint hospital for the purpose of determining the amounts payable by each of the contributing authorities. They have made an Order (2nd June, 1903) for this latter purpose.

A County Council, however, if they make a contribution to the funds of an isolation hospital (see § 21, I. H. Act, 1893, and § 2, I. H. Act, 1901) may make it a condition of contributing that the accounts of the hospital are kept in a prescribed form, and forms have been drawn up for this purpose by Dr S. Barwise, County Medical Officer of Health for Derbyshire.

Classification of expenses. The expenses of an isolation hospital may conveniently be classified, as in § 17, I. H. Act, into structural, establishment, and patients' expenses. " Structural expenses " are the original cost of providing the hospital, and include :

Preliminary expenses in formation of the hospital district.
Cost of site and expenses of local inquiries.
Cost of hospital buildings.
Cost of furnishing.
Permanent extensions.
Drainage works.
Structural repairs.

" Establishment expenses " are the cost of keeping the hospital in a state fit for the reception of patients, and include :

Ordinary repairs, painting and cleaning.
Renewal and keeping in order of appliances and furniture.
Supply of new appliances and furniture.
Salaries of doctors, nurses and servants.
All other expenses of maintaining the hospital.

Structural and establishment expenses are payable out of a common fund to which the constituent authorities of a joint district contribute on a scale fixed in the Order forming the district, usually on a basis either of assessable value or of population (see Chapter IV, p. 64).

"Patients' expenses" are the costs incurred on behalf of patients individually, and include:

Cost of removal to hospital.

Food and stimulants.

Medicine.

Disinfecting, etc.

Burial expenses.

"Special patients' expenses" are the special charge made to patients who are provided at their own desire with accommodation of an exceptional character. These are recoverable from the patient or his estate. Otherwise patients' expenses are recoverable, in the case of paupers from the guardians, and in the case of a non-pauper patient from the sanitary authority of the district from which he is sent[1]. In the case of patients from outside the hospital district an additional charge may be made as a contribution to the structural and establishment expenses.

According to § 17 (3), I. H. Act, 1893, in the case of any doubt arising as to what are structural expenses, establishment expenses, or patients' expenses the decision of the hospital committee shall be conclusive. This gives scope for diversity of practice between different hospital committees; for instance as to how much of the cost of provisions should be apportioned to staff and to patients respectively. In order to secure similarity for purposes of comparison, Dr Barwise suggests that a uniform sum of 7s. 6d. per head per week should be set down for the food of the staff, and that the rest of the cost of provisions when the hospital is in use should go to patients' expenses. He has also drawn up a form of day-book for the keeping of hospital accounts, with an index showing under which heading different articles are to be entered. In some Orders constituting Joint Hospital Boards under the Public Health Act other items beyond those above mentioned are debited to patients' expenses, as medical attendance (paid by fee per case) and extra nurses

[1] The sanitary authority may recover the cost from the patient under § 132. P. H. Act, 1875. See Chapter XI.

required. In a joint hospital district it is desirable that the sum
apportioned for "patients' expenses" should be so fixed as to
coincide as nearly as possible with the actual cost of patients'
maintenance, without leaving any large balance on either the
debit or credit side. A charge per patient fixed too high will
tend to deter constituent authorities from sending in cases, while
one fixed too low may encourage the too free use of the
hospital, which may thus come to be filled with slight cases
at a time when it is needed for serious emergencies.

Contributions by County Council.

A County Council may, where they deem it expedient for
the benefit of the county, contribute a capital or annual sum
towards the structural and establishment expenses of an isolation
hospital. They may similarly contribute to a hospital provided
under the Public Health Act, whether within the county or not,
but the consent of the Local Government Board is required to an
annual contribution by a County Council to a hospital erected,
or permanently extended by expenditure paid otherwise than
out of a loan.

Several County Councils have by a system of contributions
acquired a useful power of supervision over the isolation hospital
provision in their counties. The Essex County Council has
adopted a graduated system of contributions, giving points for
the efficiency of the hospital in various respects. A contribution
should be "per bed space" of 2000 cubic feet or other approved
amount, rather than "per bed," as the latter might encourage
local authorities to overcrowd their hospitals by putting in more
beds than they should properly contain, with a view to getting a
larger grant.

Figures of actual cost of hospitals. Some useful informa-
tion on this point is given by Dr Barwise in his Report on the
Isolation Hospitals of Derbyshire, 1906, already mentioned.
A large part of this county is provided with hospital accommo-
dation by six Hospital Committees under the Isolation Hospitals
Acts, who possess between them 10 hospitals, of which two are
for small-pox only, while in one large district, that of North
Derbyshire, there are three hospitals for other diseases in different

parts of the district; see table on p. 246. These hospitals contain in all 234 beds, and received in the year 1905 1023 patients, of whom 109 were small-pox cases. The resident staff amounted to 82 persons.

In the year 1905 the aggregate structural expenses amounted to £6417, equal to an average rate of ·95*d*. in the £, of which ·4*d*. was for structural works and ·55*d*. for repayment of loans. In individual districts the rates for structural expenses varied from ·47*d*. to 2·15*d*.; in the latter case temporary small-pox accommodation had been provided out of current rates.

Establishment expenses amounted to £7912, equal to a rate of 1·2*d*. in the £, varying in different districts from ·85*d*. to 1·82*d*.

Patients' expenses amounted to £2452, or ·36*d*. in the £, varying in different districts from ·20*d*. to ·53*d*. But as before mentioned, the method of distribution of costs between the two last headings varied in different districts, so that the figures are not comparable.

The aggregate rate over the whole area was 2·4*d*. in the £, and Dr Barwise thinks that the normal total expenditure will equal a rate of from 1½*d*. to 2½*d*. until the loans are paid off.

Correcting the establishment expenses on a uniform basis, as a rate per occupied bed space of 2000 cubic feet per annum, Dr Barwise gives figures for eight hospitals ranging from £47 to £107, the average being £74. The corrected cost per occupied bed space per annum of rations, salaries and uniforms of staff varied from £29 to £76, the average being £47.

Reckoned as cost per patient, the patients' expenses corrected on a uniform basis as regards cost of provisions averaged £1. 16*s*. per head, ranging in the eight hospitals from £1. 9*s*. 1*d*. to £2. 1*s*. 9*d*. Of the £1. 16*s*., provisions cost £1. 2*s*. 1*d*., the remainder being for costs of removal, medicine and disinfectants.

The average cost per head per annum at seven hospitals of provisions of different kinds was: Meat, fish, poultry, etc., £4·48; butter, cheese, bacon and groceries, £4·04; milk and eggs, £2·56; bread and flour, £1·03; vegetables, £0·70. Total £12·81, or 4*s*. 11*d*. per head per week.

The total amounts refunded to seven hospital committees were: by guardians £109, as "special patients' expenses" £170, out of a total amount of £2515, patients' expenses.

The salaries of the staff at the several hospitals range as follows: *Resident:* Superintendent nurse, £30 to £70. Nurses, £20 to £30. Probationers, £10 to £25. Wardmaids, £14 to £20. Domestics, £13 to £39. *Non-resident:* Clerk, £20 to £60. Medical Superintendent, £30 to £105[1].

The annual cost of maintaining isolation hospitals varies in different areas. Dr Chalmers of Glasgow has stated that the estimated outlay on isolation for 1920 in 4 large cities was respectively 3*s*. 5*d*., 3*s*. 1*d*., 1*s*. 11*d*. and 1*s*. 3*d*. per head of the population. Of course the cost depends on the volume of infectious disease in the city and the local fashion as regards isolating cases.

BIBLIOGRAPHY

Parsons. Hospital Report, 1912, and appended Memorandum on the cost of Isolation Hospitals, by B. T. Kitchin, Architect to L.G.B.
Memorandum of the Architect and the Medical Officer of the L.G.B. on inexpensive construction of Sanatoria. See appendix to Chapter XVIII.
Barwise, S., M.D. Reports on the Isolation Hospitals of Derbyshire, 1906 and 1913.
Hospital Return. 1895.
Stott, H. Draft scheme of Hospital Accounts. Public Health, Sept., 1909.
Chalmers. Transactions of the Epidemiological Section of the Royal Society of Medicine for 1920.

CHAPTER XVIII

SANATORIA FOR TUBERCULOSIS

THE various purposes for which the hospital or institutional treatment of patients with pulmonary tuberculosis has been practised have been mentioned in Chapter II, p. 43. The present chapter deals with the construction of places intended mainly for the first of those purposes, viz. the cure or arrest of the disease in cases in the early stage. Such places usually go by the name of "sanatoria," a name originally meaning "places of healing" but now specially applied to places for the treatment of tuberculosis.

What may be regarded as the earliest special institution in this country for the treatment of tuberculous patients, the Royal

[1] These are pre-war salaries.

Sea-Bathing Hospital, Margate, was established in 1791. Other early institutions of the kind are the Royal Hospital for Diseases of the Chest, City Road, London, 1814, Brompton Hospital for Consumption, 1841, Western Hospital for Incipient Consumption, Torquay, 1850, and the City of London Hospital for Diseases of the Chest, Victoria Park, 1851, and others are mentioned by Dr Bulstrode in his official report. But the methods of treatment in vogue at the time when these earlier hospitals were founded were very different from those adopted in modern sanatoria. Thus Dr J. S. Bristowe and Mr T. Holmes in their report in 1863, to which reference is made in Chapter I, while deprecating special fever hospitals, say "Hospitals for consumption are probably beneficial in treating a class of cases which require a higher and more uniform temperature than is quite consistent with the free ventilation which seems necessary for the salubrity of a general hospital for acute diseases."

Although earlier writers had recommended an open air life for consumptives, the principles of open air treatment were first clearly set out and reduced to practice in 1840 by Mr George Bodington of Sutton Coldfield, near Birmingham, who started an establishment for the purpose; but his views were not accepted at the time in England and his sanatorium was eventually turned into a lunatic asylum. His views however took root in Germany, and were developed by Brehmer, Dettweiler, Walther and others, and before the end of the century a large number of sanatoria had been erected in that country. In England no private sanatorium in the modern sense existed prior to 1898, and no "public" sanatorium, *i.e.* provided by public or private charity, by the State or by local authorities or associations, before 1899; but from that time their number has steadily increased.

A full account of the public sanatoria erected in England and Wales up to 1908 is given in Dr Bulstrode's Report to the Local Government Board "On Sanatoria for Consumption, and certain other aspects of the Tuberculosis question" published in 1908.

At that date few local authorities had made provision of the kind directly, though Birmingham had secured a site on the

Cotswolds near Cheltenham, and Bristol as well as some other authorities had purchased beds in the Winsley Sanatorium. Two boards of guardians had provided sanatoria for pauper patients on sites apart from the workhouse, and others had made adaptations or extensions of the workhouse buildings, for the purpose of treating phthisis cases. The greater number of sanatoria then in existence however had been provided through charity, by associations, or by private enterprise.

In July, 1912 sanatorium benefit under the National Insurance Act came into force, and from that time County Councils and Borough Councils began to erect sanatoria for the treatment of cases of pulmonary tuberculosis. The movement for providing proper accommodation in sanatoria for tuberculosis patients is still undergoing a process of evolution, and it is possible that the arrangements mentioned in this chapter may eventually be replaced by others of a still more advanced kind. Appended to this chapter will be found a Memorandum on provision of New Residential Institutions for the Treatment of Pulmonary Tuberculosis, issued by the late Local Government Board and dated February 1914. The plans mentioned in that Memorandum have not been reproduced here as they have apparently been superseded by others of a newer sort. On page 223 will be found a plan for a pavilion with 88 beds in a sanatorium showing the sleeping arrangements; on page 224 is shown a plan of a dining hall and kitchen for a sanatorium, with room for extension if required. These plans have been prepared in the Department of the Chief Architect of the Ministry of Health, and dated September 1920; they are reproduced here by permission.

Different arrangements are necessary for the treatment of sufferers from pulmonary tuberculosis in its various stages, *e.g.* for "early" "middle" and "advanced" cases, either in sanatoria, hospitals or combined institutions.

Sanatoria[1] are of value especially for the treatment of "early" cases, and for educational treatment of the more favourable of the "middle" cases. The sanatoria are usually situated in a country district, but they should not be too remote from a reasonably convenient railway service, otherwise difficulties in administration are liable to occur.

[1] See also p. 43 on the utility of Sanatoria.

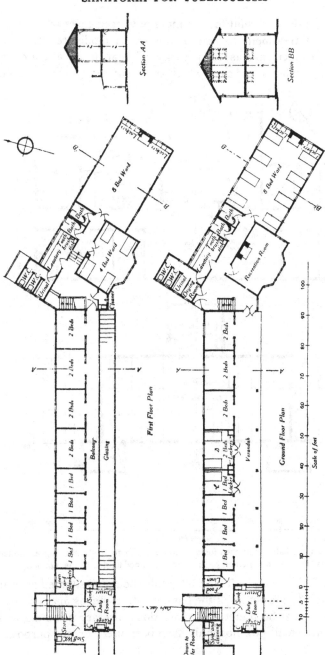

Figs. 28 and 29. Plans of ground floor and first floor of a two-storeyed pavilion for a sanatorium. Reproduced by permission of the Ministry of Health.

Hospitals are useful for the more advanced cases which need periods of treatment to restore them to a moderate degree of working capacity at least temporarily. They are useful also for very acute and far advanced cases which are a source of danger to others

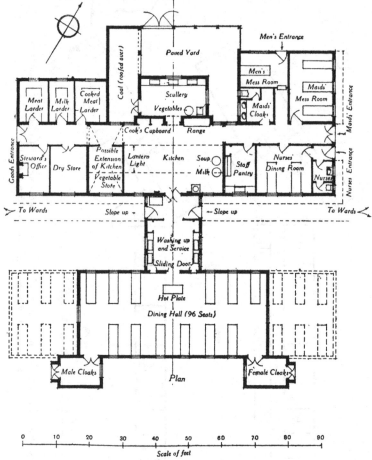

Fig. 30. Dining hall and kitchen for a sanatorium with 100 beds, showing, by dotted lines, how extension could be made to accommodate double the number.

in the patient's home. These hospitals should be situated as near as possible to the homes of the patients. In some instances special pavilions have been erected at infectious diseases hospitals, and sometimes small-pox hospitals have been used for this purpose.

Accommodation for the observation of patients with a view to definite diagnosis or the determination of the best form of treatment suited to the case, should be provided near the homes of the people ; such provision is not infrequently made in connection with the special hospital pavilions.

Combined institutions are those in which all of the above classes of cases can be treated (see plan, p. 226). Obviously they should be situated near to, and readily accessible from, a town, as for example that at Cottingham near Hull. For further details as regards sanatoria, hospitals and combined institutions for tuberculous patients see official memorandum on p. 237.

Existing hospital accommodation should be utilised as far as may be feasible. Where the accommodation is insufficient it is better to provide the additional beds required by enlargement of existing institutions rather than by the erection of new and special buildings. Advanced cases of pulmonary tuberculosis may be treated in special blocks or pavilions on the site of an existing isolation hospital, but the portion so used must be fenced off or separated from the rest of the site. The Ministry of Health only approves of the treatment of pulmonary tuberculosis in general hospitals if the bacilli are not present in the sputum, or when the case is admitted for observation or in an emergency, *e.g.* haemoptysis.

The allocation of cases of tuberculosis to the sanatorium, the hospital, or for home treatment will be the function of the " tuberculosis officer" at the " tuberculosis dispensary." The tuberculosis dispensary is not, as its name might suggest, merely a place where medicine is supplied ; its functions are as follows:

(1)   Receiving house and centre of diagnosis.

(2)   Clearing house and centre for observation.

(3)   Centre for curative treatment to a limited extent.

(4)   Centre for the examination of " contacts."

(5)   Centre for " after-care."

(6)   Information bureau and educational centre.

The tuberculosis officer should be in touch on the one hand with medical practitioners, and on the other hand with the sanatoria and hospitals providing treatment, and he should have a few beds at his disposal for purposes of observation and treatment.

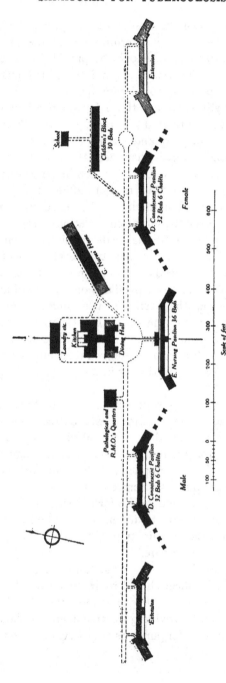

Fig. 31. Typical site plan for a combined institution for 130 beds with 12 châlets (sanatorium).

At the dispensary the following accommodation is generally desirable : an office, general waiting-room, consulting rooms (one or more) and dressing rooms. There should be facilities for laryngoscopical and bacteriological examinations and for the provision of drugs. This accommodation may commonly be obtained by the adaptation and equipment of an existing house, or again the dispensary may form a department of an existing hospital. In a few large centres, more especially where medical training is given, it may be advisable to have a special building on a larger scale. The dispensary should be easy of access to the working class population, and in county areas, in addition to the main dispensary in the most convenient available town, it will probably be found necessary to establish branch dispensaries in other towns, and local centres in the smaller towns and larger villages, at which the tuberculosis officer and nurse would attend at stated times.

In their Final Report, issued March 1913, the Departmental Committee on Tuberculosis say that they have little to add to their recommendations in the Interim Report with reference to the treatment of persons suffering from tuberculosis.

As regards prevention they point out that methods for this purpose may be divided into two classes :

(1) Those whose object is to prevent the entrance of tubercle bacilli into the human system.

(2) Those whose object is to prevent persons into whose system tubercle bacilli have entered from developing active disease.

Among measures of the first class the most important are the elimination of tubercle bacilli from food and the prevention of the spread of infection by persons already suffering from the disease. One of the principal sources of danger at the present time is the existence of a number of persons in the more acute and advanced stage of the disease who are living in that intimate contact with their families and neighbours necessitated by the ordinary conditions of their lives. "The Committee desire, therefore, to recommend as an effective means of preventing the spread of the disease, the compulsory isolation of certain cases which are in a state of high infectivity, particularly in those instances where the patients' surroundings are such as to increase the risk of other persons becoming infected. At the same time they desire to recommend that isolation should be carried out with all possible regard to the feelings of the patients and of their families and friends, and that any powers of compulsory isolation and detention possessed by or hereafter to be conferred upon local authorities should be exercised with discrimination, and only after those authorities are satisfied on thorough enquiry that the public interest requires them to be enforced in the particular instances under consideration. So far as may be practicable patients should not be removed to places difficult of access from their homes, and arrangements should be made to facilitate visits from their families and friends."

Although in the past it has been found that in many of the patients applying for sanatorium treatment for pulmonary tuberculosis the disease had made considerable advance, it may be expected that, in future, improvements in diagnosis, the notification and searching out of cases through the agency of "tuberculosis dispensaries" and the facilities afforded under the National Insurance Act for obtaining sanatorium treatment[1], will lead to a larger proportion of the patients coming under treatment in an early stage. Between such cases and those of the acute infectious diseases there are marked differences, which bear upon the character of the accommodation required.

(1)   Early "closed" cases of tuberculosis, without expectoration or discharge, are not infectious.

(2)   Patients in this stage are usually not seriously ill, as regards their present condition.

------

[1] "Sanatorium benefit" under the National Insurance Act, 1911, includes treatment not only in a "sanatorium" in the restricted sense of an institution suitable for cases in an early stage, but also in a hospital or at the patient's own home, as the circumstances of the case may require. Insured persons cannot claim sanatorium treatment as a matter of right but must be recommended for "sanatorium benefit" by the appropriate Insurance Committee. By the National Insurance Act, 1920, Sanatorium Benefit ceased on May 1st 1921, from which date Insurance Committees no longer had the duty of providing treatment for insured persons suffering from tuberculosis, except in so far as medical attendance is provided as part of Medical Benefit under the National Insurance Act of 1911. The effect of the termination of Sanatorium Benefit is that institutional treatment for tuberculosis will be provided by local Authorities for insured persons, not by arrangement with Insurance Committees but direct, as for the remainder of the population under the schemes for the institutional treatment of tuberculosis in aid of which grants are paid by the Minister of Health.

(3) The treatment needed for such cases differs materially from that of the acute infectious diseases.

A "sanatorium" therefore is not, or not so much, a place for isolating the infectious or for tending the helpless sick, but rather a place for the arrest of the disease in its early stages by removing the patient from injurious surroundings and placing him under careful medical supervision and a regimen calculated to increase his bodily powers of resistance. This regimen will include an abundant supply of pure air and light, a sufficiency of nourishing food and regulated amounts of rest and exercise as the patient's state may require. With this will be joined instruction in the rules of life necessary for the restoration and maintenance of his own health as well as for the safety of those with whom he is brought into contact.

The power to provide sanatoria is included in the powers which sanitary authorities possess under § 131, P. H. Act, 1875, to provide hospitals or temporary places for the reception of the sick. The Isolation Hospitals Acts as they stand relate only to the diseases mentioned in the Infectious Diseases Notification Acts, but can be extended to tuberculosis by an Order of the County Council with the consent of the Ministry of Health. County Councils as has been said can provide Sanatoria under the National Insurance Act, 1911.

The amount of accommodation required for sanatorium treatment was estimated by the Departmental Committee on Tuberculosis as one bed for every 5000 inhabitants in addition to hospital accommodation for advanced cases, and for educational and observational purposes. This estimate has, however, been largely exceeded in some areas. As phthisical patients in the early stage are able to travel, the area served by a sanatorium may be an extensive one and the advantages of combination of districts set out in Chapter IV will hold good[1]. In particular

---

[1] For the purpose of facilitating cooperation amongst local authorities for the provision of sanatoria and other institutions for the treatment of tuberculosis, the Local Government Board (now Ministry of Health) are empowered by § 64 (3), National Insurance Act, 1911, to make by order such provisions as appear to them necessary or expedient, by the constitution of joint committees, joint boards or otherwise, for the exercise of the authorities' powers in relation thereto, and for the apportionment of expenses between them.

such combination will facilitate the securing of a senior medical superintendent of special qualifications at an adequate salary. The Departmental Committee on Tuberculosis recommend that a sanatorium should contain not fewer than 100 beds, and that the unit area should generally be the County, County Borough or in some cases a group of Counties and County Boroughs. Moreover in a wide area there will be a greater choice of sites.

Although good results have been obtained from open air treatment even in towns, the site of a sanatorium should preferably be in an upland situation with a south slope on a dry permeable soil, in a pure and dry air, but sheltered from the prevailing winds. Sites on the tertiary gravels and sands, the lower greensand, great oolite, new red sandstone or carboniferous limestone have been chosen for many existing sanatoria. Sites on a clay soil, in damp situations and in the bottoms of valleys are liable to fogs and should be avoided. Several of the earlier hospitals for consumption are on the seacoast, but seaside sites are not now especially in favour for sanatoria for phthisis though cases of surgical tuberculosis do well there. Mountain sites are not suitable in this country, as their climate is wet and misty. The best climate is that which will allow the patients to spend most of their time in the open air. Proximity to sources of atmospheric dust, as high roads and arable ground on a loose sandy soil, should be avoided. To prevent dust the surface of the ground in the neighbourhood of the sanatorium may be covered with grass or heather.

Facilities for water supply and drainage and accessibility from a railway station should receive consideration. The area of the site should be ample in order to allow facilities for exercise and employment of patients; half an acre per patient is recommended by the Departmental Committee, but during recent years even larger sites have been purchased.

The sanatoria described by Dr Bulstrode were of very varied kinds; some were existing houses converted; others were temporary buildings in connection with an existing house which served for administration purposes; others again were specially designed buildings, sometimes of very elaborate and costly construction. The latter were establishments which had been erected by the munificence of private individuals, but Dr Bulstrode says, "Obviously the smaller the cost, the greater the number of consumptive patients who for a given sum can be accorded the advantages of sanatorium treatment; and from a purely economical standpoint, as well as from a humanitarian point of view, this is the object to be aimed at. For the most part consumption is a disease of the poorer classes who in the ordinary routine of their lives have not in the past been accustomed to anything approaching the luxuries of existence. Hence they are not likely at a sanatorium to miss things of which they have had practically no experience." He points out also that in a room constantly traversed by a copious current of fresh air the amount of cubic space per bed need not be so great as in a hospital ward ; and that the objection to wooden buildings on the ground of their inflammability and the danger to life in case of fire has not the same force in one-storey buildings for early cases, with easy means of escape from each room, as in wards for bed-ridden patients. Moreover, arrangements which are still to some extent in an experimental stage would be stereotyped by the erection of costly permanent buildings. In buildings designed as sanatoria the typical plan at first was a building consisting of two wings united by a central block containing a dining hall, the administrative departments being in this centre block or in another annexed to the rear. The building as a whole faces south. The wings may be in one line, or may be inclined to one another at an obtuse angle, so that the east wing faces S.S.W. and the west wing S.S.E. Each wing consists of a row of small wards, for one or two beds each, with a verandah in front, and a corridor behind connecting the wards, and giving access to the sanitary annexes. Each ward is furnished with permanently open means of ventilation, both back and front. In buildings of brick or stone the wings may be two storeys in height, the arrangement being repeated on the upper storey, but in wooden buildings they are only one storey high.

The Benenden Sanatorium (see Fig. 32), Kent, a two-storey building, is built on the Frazzi system. The foundations are of concrete, and the walls of hollow slabs of an artificial stone, jointed with mortar and supported at the corners with vertical iron stanchions. The total thickness of the outside walls is a little under

5 inches. It is stated that the cost of this method of construction is much less than that of brickwork as the foundations required are lighter; it can be rapidly constructed, it is warm in winter and cool in summer, and it is fireproof.

If the small wards are made, for the sake of economy, to hold two beds each, it is well to have also a few single bed wards for special cases. There may also be a larger ward for febrile cases which are confined to bed. In addition to the wards shelters are often provided in which patients may lie by day practically in the open air. See Figs. 38, 39 and 40.

The buildings should be planned with a view to expansion, and should be so arranged that separate treatment can be pro-

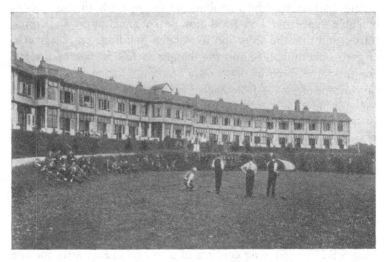

Fig. 32. Showing frontage of a part of the two-storeyed building of the National Sanatorium, Benenden, Kent, referred to on page 231.

vided for men and women. The Tuberculosis Committee also consider that it is desirable that distinct institutions, or at least separate pavilions, should be provided for children.

On p. 226 is given a typical site plan for a combined institution for 130 beds with 12 châlets. On p. 223 is shown a plan of a two-storeyed pavilion with 88 beds, and on p. 224 is given a plan of a dining hall and kitchen for a sanatorium with 100 beds. These plans, reproduced by permission of the Ministry of Health, were prepared in the Chief Architect's Department and are dated September 1920.

For further particulars the reader may be referred to Dr Bulstrode's report, and to the Local Government Board's Memorandum of 1914 appended to this chapter.

The illustration below, Fig. 33, shows a sanatorium building of Doecker construction, "strong" type—see Chapter VIII—supplied by the Hygienic Constructions and Portable Buildings, Ltd, Stockholm Road, South Bermondsey.

A sanatorium designed by Messrs Boulton and Paul of Norwich is shown in Figs. 36 and 37. It has accommodation for 12 patients along with the necessary offices; it is constructed mainly of wood and erected on brick piers, the cost being comparatively small.

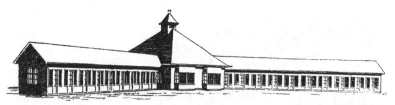

Fig. 33. Elevation of part of a sanatorium pavilion of Doecker construction for 20 beds. The administration buildings are not shown.

During recent years army huts have been converted satisfactorily for use as sanatorium buildings yielding good accommodation at a reasonable cost. Converted army huts have been erected at various sanatoria to form training sections for ex-service men needing treatment for pulmonary tuberculosis and at the same time training in a new occupation. At Wolsingham, in the county of Durham, army huts are being utilised at the County Council's Sanatorium, see Figs. 34 and 35. Each hut is 60 feet long and 15 wide, accommodating 9 patients each of whom has 64 square feet of floor space; the distance between the centres of any two beds is 8 feet measured along the wall behind the heads of the beds. A half screen separates each group of 3 beds (see Fig. 35).

As experience accumulates, changes occur in the views held

as to the construction and arrangement of Sanatoria. From time to time memoranda were issued on the subject by the late Local Government Board. The last of these is dated February 1914 (see copy appended): it is entitled Memorandum on provision of New Residential Institutions for the treatment of Pulmonary Tuberculosis. It is not improbable that another memorandum of the kind will be issued before long by the Ministry of Health.

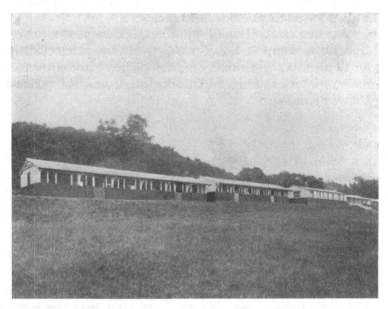

Fig. 34. Showing army huts converted for the use of ex-service men needing treatment for pulmonary tuberculosis and at the same time training in a new occupation, at the Durham County Council's Sanatorium, Wolsingham.

The plans which accompanied the 1914 memorandum have not been reproduced here.

Shelters. On pages 238 and 240 (Figs. 38, 39 and 40) are given illustrations of shelters made by Messrs Boulton and Paul, Norwich, for use in connection with the open air treatment of tuberculosis. The advantage of a revolving shelter is that it can be turned so as to screen the patient from hot sun or cold wind.

BIBLIOGRAPHY

Bulstrode, H. T.   Report to Local Government Board "On Sanatoria for Consumption, and certain other aspects of the Tuberculosis question." 1908.   (Cd. 3657.)

Interim Report of the Departmental Committee on Tuberculosis.   1912.

Final Report of the Departmental Committee on Tuberculosis.   1913.

Memorandum of Local Government Board "On the construction and arrangement of inexpensive buildings for Tuberculous patients."   1914.

Designs for the King's Sanatorium.   Lancet, Jan. 3, 1903.

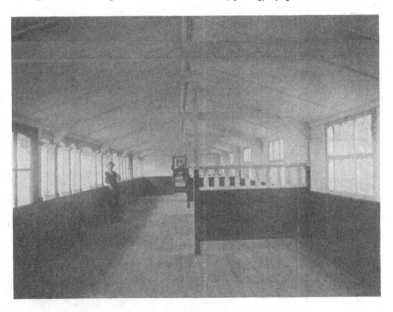

Fig. 35.   Showing interior of converted army huts used by ex-service men at the Durham County Council's Sanatorium Wolsingham.   Each hut accommodating 9 patients has two screens projecting halfway across the hut and dividing it into 3 separate sections with 3 patients in each.

Foulerton and Cole.   A Model Sanatorium for the treatment of Pulmonary Tuberculosis.   Public Health, March, 1903.

Pringle, A. M. N.   The Tuberculosis Campaign in Ipswich (with plans of Ipswich Sanatorium).   Public Health, Dec., 1911.

Davies, Sidney.   Garden shelters for Home treatment of Consumption. (Illustrated.)   Public Health, Jan., 1912.

Lister, T. D.   The treatment of Phthisis by Industrial Insurance, with special reference to the Benenden Sanatorium.   Public Health, May, 1911.

National Insurance Act, 1911.

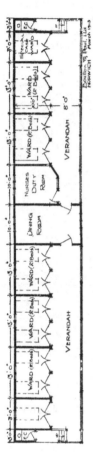

Fig. 36. Showing plan of sanatorium building for 12 patients (Messrs Boulton and Paul, Norwich), for elevation of which see Fig. 37.

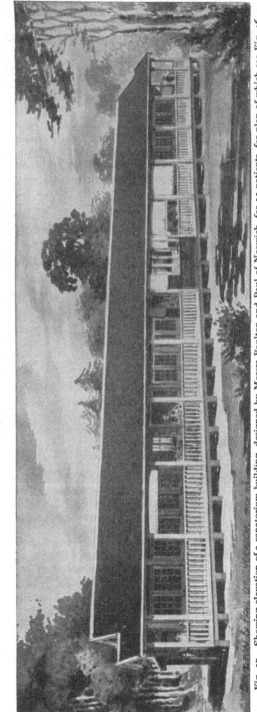

Fig. 37. Showing elevation of a sanatorium building, designed by Messrs Boulton and Paul of Norwich, for 12 patients, for plan of which see Fig. 36.

APPENDIX

MEMORANDUM ON PROVISION OF NEW RESIDENTIAL INSTITUTIONS FOR THE TREATMENT OF PULMONARY TUBERCULOSIS.

In a previous memorandum, dated the 25th February, 1913, it was indicated in a general way how nexpensive sanatorium accommodation for tuberculous persons could be erected within a comparatively short period in order to meet any pressing need in a particular locality.

The present memorandum has been prepared with a view to affording local authorities and others further assistance in the provision of special residential institutions in connection with permanent schemes for the treatment of Pulmonary Tuberculosis. The unit taken in setting out the details has been 100 beds in buildings, with 10 additional beds in shelters. For institutions containing a larger number of beds, *see* the second paragraph on page 243.

Economy in building.

In preparing this memorandum, economy has been borne in mind throughout, but, it is believed, without any sacrifice of efficiency. The cost of an institution—apart from the cost and the character of the site—depends primarily on its planning; after this on the character of the materials used in its construction. The local circumstances must be taken into account in determining the choice of building materials.

Site.

In the selection of a site the most important considerations to be taken into account are—

(1) Area.
(2) Elevation in relation to surrounding country.
(3) Cheerfulness of outlook.
(4) Protection from certain winds.
(5) Subsoil.
(6) Drainage facilities.
(7) Water supply.
(8) Convenience of access.

(1) The area of land required for the site will depend upon the number of patients and the type of cases.

The site of a sanatorium should be sufficiently large to permit of open-air employment of a considerable number of patients. It is desirable that a site of 50 acres in extent should be provided for 100 patients if land is readily available and the cost is low, but an area of not less than 20 acres may suffice for this number of patients where suitable land is difficult to obtain or the

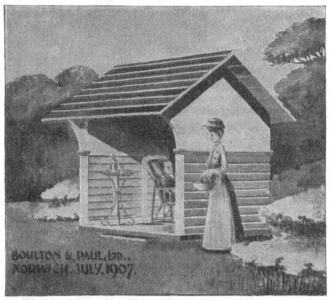

Fig. 38.   Showing a revolving shelter accommodating two patients.

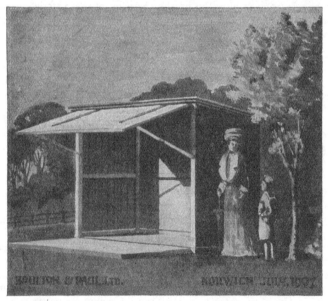

Fig. 39.   Showing wooden shelter; the whole front can be closed when not in use.

cost of land is high. It is desirable that in all cases an area of at least one-fifth of an acre should be allowed per patient.

(2), (3), and (4) The site should preferably slope gradually to the south and be protected on the north and east by high ground, preferably wooded. In some districts protection from westerly and south-westerly gales may be desirable. The site should be moderately elevated above the country lying to the south of it.

(5) The subsoil has importance, not only as regards dampness or dryness, but also because the cost of building may depend somewhat upon its character. The main consideration is that the site should be dry. This must be secured if necessary by proper drainage, but a site requiring extensive drainage should, as a rule, be avoided.

(6) If drainage into a public sewer is impracticable, the site should be suitable for the provision of an adequate sewage disposal system.

(7) It will be necessary to ascertain that an abundant supply of pure water is available.

(8) The site should, if possible, be within easy reach of a railway station. The cost of carriage from the station to the site will form an important factor, not only as regards construction, but also in the subsequent maintenance of the institution. There is the further consideration that it is undesirable that patients who are acutely ill should be unduly remote from their relatives.

Buildings.

In residential institutions for the treatment of pulmonary tuberculosis the following provision will be required:

(1) Patients' sleeping accommodation.

(2) Kitchen, dining hall, and offices.

(3) Staff block containing quarters for Resident Medical Officer, Matron, and Staff.

(4) Out-buildings, including laundry, boiler house, disinfector, sputum destructor, mortuary, etc.

General Considerations as to Accommodation for Patients.

As the planning of the institution will depend on the stage of disease of the tuberculous patients proposed to be admitted to it, it is necessary to set out a classification of cases of pulmonary tuberculosis arranged from the standpoint of accommodation in residential institutions.

Group A. *Cases in which permanent improvement or recovery may usually be anticipated.*

Group B. *Cases in which only temporary, though possibly prolonged, improvement may be anticipated.*

Such cases will include:

(1) Patients who may be expected to recover considerable ability to work, as a result of protracted treatment.

(2)   Patients admitted for a short term for educational treatment.

(3)   Patients with advanced disease, many of whom improve greatly under institutional treatment.

Group C.   *Advanced cases requiring continuous medical care and nursing.*

Group D.   *Cases requiring special observation.*

(1)   Patients admitted for the purpose of diagnosis.

(2)   Patients needing to be watched, before the best form of continued treatment can be determined.

"Emergency" cases, *e.g.*, patients with hæmoptysis, etc., may come within any of the above groups.

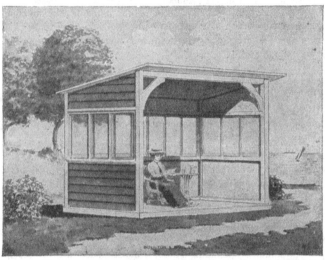

Fig. 40.   Showing wooden shelter which can be mounted on revolving gear
at a comparatively small extra expense.

For the sake of clearness, the term *sanatorium* is used hereafter to indicate an institution mainly devoted to the reception of patients in Group A, the term *hospital* to indicate an institution provided for the reception of patients in Groups B, C, and D, and the term *combined institution* to indicate an institution devoted to the reception of patients in all four groups.

Very commonly, however, patients in Group B (1) are treated in institutions intended for patients in Group A; but the advantage of the protracted treatment of patients in the former group in a *sanatorium* is somewhat doubtful. Occasionally patients in Group D may be received into a *sanatorium*, but such patients are usually better treated in a *hospital*, situated nearer the patient's home than the *sanatorium*, when both institutions are available.

The patients in all four groups may be treated in a *combined institution*, in separate rooms or pavilions. This arrangement is most suitable for areas with a population too small to require the provision of 100 beds for patients in Group A. A *combined institution* should be so situate as to secure fairly easy access of relatives to patients acutely ill, while giving good local conditions for patients in Group A.

Children's Pavilion. If it is desired to make provision for children, whether on the site of a residential institution for adults or on a different site, the Board of Education should be consulted.

Sleeping Accommodation for Patients.

The sleeping accommodation provided in residential institutions for the treatment of pulmonary tuberculosis is commonly of one or more of the following types:

I. Single-bedded rooms; II. Two-bedded rooms; III. Beds on both sides of a ward as in the ordinary isolation hospital; IV. Shelters.

I. Single rooms are often desirable for patients who require a considerable amount of nursing whether in Groups A, B, or C. These rooms should be situated in the special nursing section. Single rooms may also be required for patients in Group D. The rooms for patients in Group D need not all be situated in the special nursing block.

II. Two-bedded rooms are suitable for all types of patients with the exception of the cases referred to above for whom single rooms are required.

III. Wards will generally be found useful for patients in Group B who are able to be up and about all day. They may also be used for some of the patients in Group A. If the wards are situated near a nurse's duty room they may also be suitable for patients in Group B who require only a limited amount of nursing, and are not sufficiently ill to make the use of single-bedded rooms desirable.

IV. Shelters single or double-bedded are suitable for patients in Groups A and B who are able to be up and about all day. Single-bedded shelters may also be useful for doubtful cases sent for diagnosis (Group D (1)) and for training patients with a view to the subsequent use of shelters at home.

Shelters. Owing to difficulties in supervision and administration it is undesirable to have a large proportion of the sleeping accommodation in shelters, and as a rule provision of this kind should not exceed 10 per cent. of the total accommodation. Electric bell communication should be provided between each shelter and the nurses' duty room. These shelters may be used for training patients, about to leave the sanatorium, to sleep in shelters after their return home. It is desirable, therefore, that the shelter used should be simple in construction, and similar to those lent out for use at home.

In deciding upon the kind and the proportional amount of the different types of sleeping accommodation the following general considerations should be borne in mind:

(1) It is desirable that patients in different stages of disease should as far as practicable be treated in different wards or rooms.

(2) It is desirable, in order to secure adequate and continuous attention to patients along with economy of staff, that, so far as practicable, all patients requiring special nursing should be treated in a section of the institution devoted to this purpose.

(3) Subject to the foregoing considerations there is no administrative or other difficulty in having patients in different stages of disease in the same pavilion.

The term "nursing section or pavilion" is used throughout this memorandum to refer to that portion of the institution set aside for the treatment of those patients who are not able to be up and about all day but require a certain amount of special nursing or supervision, and the term "convalescent section or pavilion" to that portion of the institution allocated to patients who are able to be up and about all day and to take all their meals in the dining hall.

The special nursing section should be quiet and not liable to disturbance from the passing to and fro of other patients, and should be sufficiently near the central kitchen to permit easy service.

For a *sanatorium*, about 20 per cent. of the sleeping accommodation for patients should be in the special nursing section; for a *combined institution*, it is desirable that about 36 per cent. of the sleeping accommodation should be so placed.

In a *combined institution*, it is undesirable that any special pavilion or section should be used exclusively for patients with advanced disease. The pavilion or section used for these patients should also include accommodation in separate rooms for patients in Groups A, B, or D, requiring special nursing, rest in bed or supervision. If this is done patients will not be led to suppose from the place where they are being treated that their cases are hopeless.

Types of Buildings.

The drawings[1] which accompany this memorandum aim at giving an indication of the lines on which buildings for this purpose may be designed, and it is hoped that these may be of service to those who are engaged in the provision of institutions for tuberculous patients.

The following plans are appended to the memorandum[1].

A. Block plan of a 100 bed sanatorium with three separate pavilions.

B. Block plan of a 100 bed sanatorium with a single pavilion.

C. Ground plan of Staff Block.

[1] Not reproduced here, but see figs. 28 and 29.

D.   First floor plan of Staff Block.
E.   Plan of Dining hall and Kitchen Block.
F.   Plan of Nursing Pavilion for 36 beds.
G.   Plan of Convalescent Pavilion for 32 beds.
H.   Plan of two-storeyed pavilion for 100 beds.
I.   Plan of two-storeyed pavilion for 100 beds (alternative design).

It will not usually be practicable to provide in a single one-storeyed building 100 beds in rooms or wards with beds arranged on one side only. Such an arrangement would necessitate a very long building, which may be expensive to construct, except on a level site, and which would be inconvenient to administer. For an institution for 100 patients it will often be preferable to arrange for three separate pavilions (Scheme I); under some circumstances it may be found desirable to provide the accommodation in one two-storeyed building (Scheme II).

If an institution for more than 100 beds is required, it will usually be preferable to adopt a modification of Scheme I, with at least three pavilions, one a special nursing section, and two separate pavilions for males and females respectively.

Schemes I and II have both been prepared upon the assumption that equal accommodation will be required for each sex. They may require modification in this respect according to local needs.

An arrangement is also shown by which 10 beds between the duty rooms in the special nursing pavilion in Plan F and in the central section of the ground floor in Plans H and I, ordinarily intended in each instance for 5 male and 5 female patients, can be utilised either entirely for male or entirely for female patients, as occasion may require. Some elasticity in the amount of accommodation for the two sexes is thus secured.

Scheme 1.

(Details of the various blocks are given in plans C, D, E, F and G.)[1]

Scheme I has been prepared to secure the advantages to be obtained by having one pavilion for patients requiring special nursing or supervision and two additional pavilions for male and female patients respectively, who are able to be up and about all day. This arrangement makes for efficiency and economy in nursing, and secures separation of the sexes more efficiently than is possible if all patients are treated in the same building.

It has been prepared for a *combined institution*, and shows a special nursing pavilion for 36 patients, a pavilion for 32 male and a pavilion for 32 female patients. The plan can be modified so as to make it suitable for a *sanatorium*, by reducing the accommodation in the special nursing pavilion to about 20 beds and by increasing that in the separate pavilions for male and female patients.

[1] Not reproduced.

The block plan shows that the central portion of the site is occupied by the staff block, kitchen and dining hall block, and out-buildings, and by the special nursing pavilion; the eastern and western sections are occupied by the separate convalescent pavilions for male and female patients respectively. The portions of the site devoted to male and female patients are thus separated, so far as possible, by administrative and other buildings.

Special Nursing Pavilion (*Plan F*). For convenience of service this pavilion is connected with the centrally situated kitchen and dining hall block by a covered way about 60 feet in length. The plans show a central service kitchen. On either side of this kitchen is provided a nurse's duty room and accommodation for 10 patients in four double-bedded and two single-bedded rooms. It is intended that this central section should be used for those patients who are acutely ill. The north verandah will be useful for nurses attending on the patients. At the end of this verandah a hospital slop sink has been provided. It is desirable that arrangements should be made for heating some of these bedrooms.

At each end of these centrally situated rooms is a lavatory section; and, beyond this, in the wings is accommodation for those patients who require only a moderate amount of nursing. This accommodation may be provided either in double-bedded rooms or in small wards. The latter arrangement is shown on Plan F.

The section between the service kitchen and the duty room on each side is practically cut off from the section beyond the duty room. A small lavatory annexe situated behind the service kitchen, and containing two w.c.'s and one bath room, has been provided for these sections. This arrangement makes it possible to use these sections entirely for male or entirely for female patients or for five patients of each sex. In the event of the sections being occupied by patients of different sexes, each section would have a separate w.c., but the bath room would be common to the two.

Convalescent Pavilions (*Plan G*). The sleeping accommodation is shown partly in double-bedded rooms and partly in a small ward. As patients occupying these pavilions will be able to take their meals in the dining hall no provision has been made for the service of food, and the pavilions need not be situated close to the central kitchen block. No provision has been made in these pavilions for special nursing, as it is assumed that patients requiring this will be transferred to the special nursing pavilion.

SCHEME II.

(Details of the various blocks are given in plans C, D, E, H and I.)[1]

Plans of a two-storeyed building have been prepared to meet those cases where local circumstances make it desirable to provide the whole of the sleeping accommodation for patients in a single building. The plans have

---

[1] Not reproduced.

been prepared for a *sanatorium*. If it is proposed to use such a two-storeyed building as a *combined institution*, the plan can be modified to secure more accommodation on the ground floor, within the special nursing section.

Provision has been made for a centrally situated special nursing section on the ground floor. The general arrangement of this section is similar to that of the special nursing pavilion included in Scheme I. Arrangements have been made for the accommodation of patients needing little nursing supervision on the first floor and in the wings on the ground floor. As it is suggested that the first floor shall be used only by patients who are able to be up and about, only narrow balconies for access to the rooms have been provided in order that the lighting and ventilation of the ground floor rooms may not be materially interfered with.

It will be noted that the plan of the first floor differs from that of the ground floor, only one duty room having been provided.

General Observations.

Space for patients and height of walls. The accommodation should be so arranged that a floor space of at least 64 square feet will be available for each patient; the distance between the centres of the heads of any two adjoining beds should not be less than eight feet measured along the wall behind the heads of the beds.

Patients' rooms should not be less than 8 feet 6 inches high; wards should be higher, but may be carried partly into the roof and ventilated by openings in the gable end.

Doors should be made on the "stable door" pattern so that in inclement weather the lower portion may be closed while the upper portion is left open. They should be constructed in the form of French casements with a clear opening of not less than 3 feet 6 inches, so that beds may easily be wheeled through them.

Windows should preferably be of the casement pattern and be hung "to fold" without mullions.

Baths should be provided on a scale of about one to twelve patients. They may be of enamelled iron and should be fitted with large taps and wastes to facilitate filling and emptying. Spray baths may also be provided.

There should be at least one water closet for every twelve patients. Hospital slop sinks should be provided in the special nursing pavilion.

Every institution should have ample storeroom accommodation for linen, clothes, etc., and lockers for boots and shoes. The provision of some arrangement for drying patients' clothes will also be advisable.

Day Shelters. The question as to whether day shelters shall be provided will require consideration for each proposed institution; if verandah accommodation is not adequate, day shelters will be needed. These should be of inexpensive construction.

Recreation Rooms. In view of the importance of continuous open air treatment of patients, it is unwise to encourage them to collect in a recreation room, except for a very limited time, or on special occasions. In view of these considerations the dining room has frequently been regarded as sufficing for the use of patients for recreation, lectures, etc. If it is considered necessary to provide special recreation rooms for use on wet days, or in winter evenings, these may conveniently be added at the ends of the pavilions for convalescent patients.

Kitchen and dining hall accommodation (Plan E). The block containing the patients' dining hall and kitchen for patients and staff should preferably be a one-storey building, which should be placed near to the administrative block and to the rooms for patients requiring special nursing. It may be connected with the special nursing pavilion, if desirable, by a covered way.

The dining hall should, if practicable, have a southerly aspect.

The consulting room, dispensary and laboratory, which should be centrally situated, may also conveniently be included in this block.

Unless other accommodation is available for the male domestic staff provision may be made for them in an upper floor of the kitchen and dining hall block above the store rooms, etc.

Staff block (Plans C and D). The position of this building should be selected with a view to giving the greatest facilities for economical service and administration. The accommodation for a sanatorium with 110 beds will include medical officer's quarters, offices, matron's quarters, dining room for nurses, bedroom accommodation for the nurses and servants. Each nurse should have a separate bedroom of an area of about 100 square feet. Usually one nurse will be required for 12 patients; but more will be needed if a considerable number of patients with advanced disease are being treated. Baths and water closets should be provided in the proportion of not less than one to each 12 nurses or servants.

It is desirable that the principal cooking for the staff should be done in the central kitchen block, so that a separate fully equipped kitchen is not required in the administrative block. A small kitchen pantry with food store is shown on the plan adjoining the nurses' dining room. This could be provided with a small range or gas cooker for minor cooking.

Out-buildings. The laundry should consist of receiving room and wash-house, drying room, and ironing and delivery room. Mortuary accommodation may be provided in the same block.

The amount of boiler house accommodation will depend on the amount of steam required for laundry, disinfector, heating and hot water supply and for driving dynamos if electric current is to be generated in this way for lighting or other purposes. Special provision should be made for the sterilisation of sputum and for the cleansing of sputum cups. Unless suitable arrangements are available elsewhere some form of disinfector for clothing and bedding should be provided.

Hot water supply. An ample and constant supply of hot water is desirable and the system should be capable of easy extension.

Heating and lighting. It will usually be unnecessary to heat the patients' quarters excepting the dining hall and some of the rooms for patients requiring special nursing. A system of low pressure hot water heating will be found most economical for this purpose.

Electric lighting should be employed where electric current is available or can be produced economically. It may be necessary to use coal gas, acetylene or petrol air gas: these illuminants have been found to be fairly satisfactory for use in sanatoria if suitable fittings are provided and adequate precautions are taken against fire.

Construction. Where, owing to local circumstances, the use of brickwork would be economical, cheap bricks may often be employed faced externally, if necessary, with rough-cast or cement. Walls in exposed positions should be of hollow construction.

In some districts other materials may be less expensive and may be employed, such as steel framing carrying terra-cotta slabs, or concrete slabs or blocks plastered internally and cemented externally, or timber-framing lined internally with asbestic sheeting or expanded metal lathing plastered with a hard setting plaster, rough-cast or coated externally with weather boarding chemically treated. The roofs should be of simple construction and may be covered with slates, tiles or asbestic material. The floors of verandahs should be of impermeable material.

ARTHUR NEWSHOLME,
Medical Officer to the Board.

BROOK KITCHIN,
Architect to the Board.

LOCAL GOVERNMENT BOARD.
February, 1914.

CHAPTER XIX

EXAMPLES OF ISOLATION HOSPITALS

TABLE I on p. 248 is taken from the Author's report on Isolation Hospitals, and gives particulars of a number of hospitals in different parts of the country, with the cost of their erection, up to 1911.

TABLE I. *Giving particulars of a number of hospitals in different parts of the country, with the cost of their erection, up to 1911.*

Hospital Authority	Situation of hospital	Area of district in acres	Population of district 1911	Area of site in acres ‡‡	Number of ward-blocks	Number of beds sanctioned	Cost of site £	Total cost of hospital £	Cost per bed with site £	Cost per bed without site £	Special points
Acton Urban District Council	Acton ...	2,305	57,523	3¾	3	33†	Original hospital —	17,420 (ex. site)	—	528	Original hospital of brick. Administration block an old house unsuitable for the purpose. Steam laid on to hospital from town destructor for heating. New block, 1911, of concrete slabs 4 inches thick, cheap, not yet in use at time of visit.
					4	69	Hospital as enlarged in 1911 —	22,070 (ex. site)	—	320	
Bridport Town Council	Pitwell, Allington, in Bridport Rural District	672	5,919	4 (3)	1	8†	690	2,490 (incl. site)	311	225	The low cost per bed of this hospital is due to its comprising a single ward-block containing a number of beds larger apparently than the borough has needed. Buildings partly of corrugated iron.
Brighouse Joint Hospital Board.	Clifton, Halifax Rural District	11,771	34,238	5	3	30†	900	12,835 (incl. site)	428	398	Very complete and well equipped ‖.
Colne and Holme Hospital Committee	Meltham ...	45,686	61,239	19 (5)	4	50†	900	23,310 (ex. site)	484	466	Very complete and well equipped ‖.
Croydon Rural and Merton Joint Hospital Board	Beddington Corner, in Carshalton Urban District	22,780	78,074*	19 (6)	5	62†	4,500	33,840 (incl. site)	546	473	Costly site. Isolation block of special cruciform design‖.
Cuckfield Rural District Council	Gate House Lane, Hurstpierpoint	54,095	16,853	14½ (part only)	3	24	1,000	13,000 (incl. site)	541	500	High cost per bed partly due to price of site, clay soil, and cost of road making, laying on water, and works of sewage disposal.
East Ham Town Council	East Ham ...	3,324	133,504	17½	Permanent 3 Temporary	58†	10,000	27,729 (incl. site)	478	306	Administration block and two pavilions of corrugated iron, erected out of current rates. Isolation block of special design containing 12 single-bed rooms.

											Remarks
Gloucester Town Council	Over, Gloucester Rural District	2,314	50,029*	24 (6½)	3	40	3,958	25,564	639	540	Site unnecessarily large, and involved much expense in laying out, road making, and sewage disposal. Details of buildings, fittings, and furniture unnecessarily elaborate and expensive.
Huddersfield Town Council	Huddersfield, 2 miles from centre of town	11,550	107,825	18	4	112† (+8 phthisis)	4,635	54,371 (incl. site)	485	444	Hospital erected by loan under local Act without Board's sanction. Construction expensive; ward-blocks built on arches, and connected by covered corridors on raised causeways. In addition to permanent buildings there is a temporary building for eight phthisis cases.
Kirkburton Isolation Hospital Committee.	Kirkburton ...	17,305	20,789	4½	2	24	292	9,988 (incl. site)	416	404	Cheap site purchased out of current rates. Ends of large wards in pavilion partitioned off to form convalescent rooms‖.
Lydd Town Council	Lydd...	12,082	2,874	½	1	6†	Belonged to Corporation	1,550	—	258	Hospital a single two-storey building, containing two 2-bed wards and kitchen on ground floor, and a 2-bed ward and rooms for staff on first floor‖.
Newport (Monmouthshire) Town Council	Allt-yr-Vn, Newport	4,504	83,700	5¼	4	54†	2,578 with some buildings	23,831 (incl. site)	441	394	Site costly, and its steepness involved extra expense in building. Separate laundry for staff provided, but found unnecessary.
Nottingham Town Council	Bagthorpe ...	10,935	259,942	12½	4	112½†	2,500	Permanent buildings 32,000 —		285	Hospital erected without Board's sanction, partly by loan under local Act of 1883, partly out of current rates. The ward-blocks are connected by enclosed brick corridors, which are used for the "open-air" treatment of patients. In addition to the permanent ward-blocks there are temporary farm buildings, used for phthisis cases.

* Patients are also received under agreement from other districts.
† The number of beds for which the hospital was designed, in accordance with the Local Government Board's standard of space, is in practice exceeded.
‡ The figures in brackets show the area enclosed to form the hospital curtilage, where the whole area is not used for hospital purposes.
‖ See plan following.

TABLE I (continued).

Hospital Authority	Situation of hospital	Area of district in acres	Population of district 1911	Area of site in acres ++	Number of ward-blocks	Number of beds sanctioned	Cost of site	Total cost of hospital	Cost per bed with site	Cost per bed without site	Special points
							£	£	£	£	
Penistone Isolation Hospital Committee	Hoyland's Moor, Hoylandswaine Urban District	34,990	18,341	4	2	14	Given to Hospital Committee	6,000 (ex. site)	—	430	Site given and hospital erected with special regard to economy, but the small number of beds involves higher cost per bed.
Rhondda Town Council	Ystrad, in Urban District	23,885	152,798	5	2	32	800	15,836 (incl. site)	495	470	Hospital has been erected in sections out of current rates, but is designed on lines similar to the Board's, and is substantially built with elaborate and costly finish and fittings. Steep site, involving much excavation.
Settle Rural District Council	Austwick, Settle Rural District	152,007	14,902	5	2	20	600	6,528 (ex. site)	356	326	Low cost of hospital due to: (1) building stone abundant in neighbourhood; (2) sewers and water service available; (3) buildings and fittings, though good and substantial, are of simple design.
Chiddingstone Isolation Hospital Committee	Hever, Sevenoaks Rural District	25,822	8,239	6 (part only)	2	12	360	6,750 (incl. site)	562	532	Ward-blocks of special design, each containing a 3-bed, 2-bed, and 1-bed ward. Site purchased out of current rates‖.
Sevenoaks Rural District Council	Otford, Sevenoaks Rural District	37,514	15,791	5	2	12†	2,600	9,300 (incl. site)	775	587	Ward-blocks similar to those at Hever Hospital. The excessive cost of this hospital as compared with Hever was due to the difficulty of obtaining a site. Administration block made large enough to serve for temporary buildings already on the site.
Stroud Joint Hospital Board	Cainscross, Stroud Rural District	39,987	39,872*	4 (3½)	4	44	650	12,538 (incl. site)	285	270	Low cost of hospital due to: (1) site cheap for building land, and sewers, water service and gas available; (2) price of building is low in the district; (3) hospital though substantially built and sufficiently equipped, is of plain and simple design and ordinary

Authority	Situation										Remarks
Tonbridge Rural District	Capel, Pembury, Tonbridge Rural District	46,853	17,771	3	1	10	300			270	Old block of brick, erected by loan in 1887.
						10†	300	2,700 (ex. site) New iron block	575 and extras	About 58–60	New block erected out of current rates, of corrugated iron lined with Eternite (asbestos) slabs, used for 16 beds. Difficulty has been found in warming it.
Tunbridge Wells, Tonbridge and Southborough Joint Small-Pox Hospital Board	Dislingbury, in Pembury in Tonbridge Rural District	53,902	75,271	10 (2½)	2	22†	700 with buildings	2,325 (incl. site)	105	—	The Joint Hospital Board were able to buy cheaply a site with existing buildings which serve for administration purposes. The ward-blocks are of temporary character and do not afford Board's standards of space per bed.
Undercliff Isolation Hospital Committee	Ventnor ...	6,542	9,058 (1901)	1¼	1	4†	leased 999 years £16 p.a	3,420 (and site)	—	855	The high cost per bed of this hospital is explained by its small size and few beds. Difficulties with water supply, for which special pumping arrangements are necessary.
Waltham Joint Hospital Board	Honey Lane; Waltham Holy Cross Urban District	16,859	38,366	10 (2)	4	40	1,400	14,850 (incl. site)	371	336	Hospital of simple design but well equipped, cost moderate.
Walthamstow Urban District Council	Chingford Urban District	4,343	124,597	19¾	4	82	2,625	42,212	515	482	A cubicle block containing 12 cells, separated from one another by glass partitions and separately approached from open air under verandahs‖. A convalescent block of special design.
West Ham ...	Plaistow ...	4,683	289,102	3¾	7	212	7,718	146,327 (incl. site)	690	637	Two-storey blocks, connected by corridors, on confined site. "Barrier system" of nursing in operation.

* Patients are also received under agreement from other districts.
† The number of beds for which the hospital was designed, in accordance with the Local Government Board's standard of space, is in practice exceeded.
‡ The figures in brackets show the area enclosed to form the hospital curtilage, where the whole area is not used for hospital purposes.
‖ See plan following.

TABLE II. *Giving particulars of Isolation Hospitals erected in Derbyshire, including Structural Details and Structural Expenses.*

A. Hospitals erected under Isolation Hospitals Act	Area of Site	Nature of Fencing	Type of Hospital	Disinfector, Laundry, Ambulance, etc.	Population served by Hospital	Area served by Hospital in acres	Rateable value of Hospital District	Amount of Loan
							£	£
Belper ...	6 acres with land lease	7 ft. galvanized iron	Brick Administrative Block, with 10 Bedrooms; S. F. Pavilion, 12 Beds; L. G. B. Observation Block, 4 Beds; Private Ward, 2 Beds, all brick; Small-pox Pavilion, 12 Beds. Galvanized iron lined with wood. Since Hospital erected, detached house built for caretaker, and covered corridors built connecting different pavilions. Public Water Supply and Gas laid on. Telephone.	Steam Disinfector (Thresh), Machine Laundry, 2-Horse Ambulance (horses hired), Mortuary, Discharging Block, consisting of Unrobing Room, Bath Room, and Dressing Room.	70,390	66,511	304,197	*7,600
Chesterfield : Penmore ...	12 a. 1 r. 13 p.	7 ft. corrugated iron	Brick Administrative Block, with 10 Bedrooms; S. F. Pavilion, 14 Beds; Enteric Block, 10 Beds; L. G. B. Observation Block, 4 Beds ; Private Ward, 2 Beds, all brick. Public Water Supply, Gas, and Telephone.	Steam Disinfector (Washington Lyons), Machine Laundry, Ambulance (horse kept), Mortuary, Discharge Block, consisting of Bath Room and 2 Dressing Rooms attached to Laundry.	47,560	15,704	144,353	11,583
Newbold (Small-pox)	5 acres	Post and rail	Corrugated iron. Caretaker's Cottage, and Pavilion to hold 12 Beds. Public Water Supply. No telephone.	Disinfector at Penmore.				
High Peak ...	8 a. 1 r. 19 p.	Stone wall, 8 ft. high	Dressed Stone Administrative Block, walls 21 ins. thick, 10 Beds; S. F. Pavilion, 12 Beds; Observation Wards, 6 Beds, all dressed stone. Small-pox Wards, 16 Beds, rough wooden buildings. Public Water Supply. Gas laid on. Telephone.	Low Pressure Current Steam Disinfector (Barwise specification), Machine Laundry, Ambulance (horse hired), 2 Mortuaries separate for Small-pox, Discharging Block consisting of Unrobing, Bath, and Dressing Rooms attached to	30,230	97,666	217,136	11,108

North Derbyshire Joint Committee: Dronfield ...	2 a. 2 r. 19 p.	Brick and stone, 8 ft. high	Brick Administrative Block, with 10 Bedrooms; S. F. Pavilion, 12 Beds; L. G. B. Observation Block, 4 Beds; Private Wards, 4 Beds, all brick. Public Water Supply. Telephone.	Steam Disinfector (Thresh), Hand Laundry, Ambulance (horses hired), Discharging Block, consisting of Unrobing Room, Bath Room, and Dressing Room.				6,698
Mastin Moor ...	3 acres	Corrugated iron, 7 ft. high	Brick Administrative Block, with 10 Bedrooms; S. F. Pavilion, 12 Beds; L. G. B. Observation Block, 4 Beds; Private Wards, 4 Beds, all brick. No telephone. Public Water Supply. Acetylene Gas Plant.	Steam Disinfector (Thresh), Hand Laundry, Ambulance (horses hired), Discharging Block, with Unrobing, Bath, and Dressing Rooms.	150,220 (Dronfield, Mastin Moor, Morton and Spital together)	120,708	594,132	6,610
Morton	6 acres	Split oak, 6 ft. 6 ins. high	Brick Administrative Block, with 10 Bedrooms; S. F. Pavilion, 12 Beds; L. G. B. Observation Block, 4 Beds; Private Wards, 2 Beds, all of brick. No telephone. Public Water Supply.	Steam Disinfector (Thresh), Hand Laundry, Ambulance (horses hired), Discharging Block with Unrobing, Bath, and Dressing Rooms attached to Laundry.				8,092
Spital ... ... (Small-pox)	6 acres	Quick set hedge	Wood and Iron Buildings. Public Water laid on. No telephone.	Disinfector at Penmore.				
Repton	4 acres	Corrugated iron, 7 ft. high	Brick Administrative Block, with 8 Bedrooms; S. F. Pavilion, 12 Beds; L. G. B. Observation Block, 4 Beds. Water Supply from well. Electric Light. Detached Cottage for Caretaker. No telephone. (See Figs. 41 and 42, pp. 250 and 251.)	Steam Disinfector (Thresh), Hand Laundry, Ambulance (horses hired).	15,277	52,856	147,802	7,645
Shardlow	5 acres	Boarded fence, 6 ft. 6 in. high	Brick Administrative Block with 8 Bedrooms; S. F. Pavilion, 12 Beds; L. G. B. Observation Block, 4 Beds; Private Ward, 2 Beds. Water Supply from well. Gas laid on. No telephone.	Low pressure current Steam Disinfector (Barwise specification), Ambulance (horse hired), Discharging Block with Unrobing, Bath, and Dressing Rooms attached to Administrative Block.	45,190	48,049	246,110	9,143

* Without Land.

TABLE II (continued).

B. Hospitals erected *not* under Isolation Hospitals Act	Area of Site	Nature of Fencing	Type of Hospital	Disinfectory, Laundry, Ambulance, etc.	Population served by Hospital	Area served by Hospital in acres	Rateable value of Hospital District	Amount of Loan
Buxton	2 acres	Rubble wall & galvanized iron, 7 ft. high	Stone Administrative Cottage, 3 Bed-rooms; 2 L. G. B. Isolation Blocks, for 10 Patients, in stone; 16 Beds in galvanized iron building. Telephone.	Steam Disinfector (Washington Lyons), Ambulance (Council's horses), Detached Laundry and Mortuary.	11,500	1,310	£91,536	£ *3,263
Haddon	¼ acre	Iron railing	Stone Hospital belonging to the Whitworth Hospital Trustees. Use of 6 Beds contracted for. Telephone.	Steam Disinfector (Bradford), no Ambulance, arrangements made with local cabproprietors, Bath in ward and final Bath in kitchen before discharge.	35,880	107,065	175,202	†5,000
Glossop Boro' ...	about 1 acre	Quick set 5 ft. high, boards 6 ft. 6 ins. high	Wood and Corrugated Iron Buildings, floor space for 10 Beds, but 32 have been accommodated. Public Water Supply. Telephone.	No Steam Disinfector, Ambulance (Corporation's own horses).	21,526	3,050	78,789	Paid out of current rate
Ilkeston Boro' ...	about 1 acre	Quick set hedge	No detached Administrative Block. Wooden Hospital. Could accommodate about 20 Patients. Public Water Supply. Telephone.	No Steam Disinfector, Ambulance kept, and horses from Town Hall.	29,250	2,526	82,402	About £1,000

* Without Land.   † £200 capitalised at 4 per cent.

Table II on p. 252 is taken from Dr Barwise's Report of 1906 on the Isolation Hospitals of Derbyshire, and gives particulars of the hospitals which have been erected in that county (excluding the county borough of Derby). Most of them have been erected through the instrumentality of the Derbyshire County Council, under the Isolation Hospital Acts. These are all of the same general type, of which the Repton Hospital at Etwall, shown in the accompanying illustrations (Figs. 41 and 42), may be taken as an example.

The following plans show some ward-blocks of special design which have been adopted at certain of the hospitals referred to in the table above, and in preceding pages.

Stroud Joint Hospital, Cainscross, Gloucestershire.

The plan of the Stroud Joint Hospital at Cainscross, Gloucestershire, shows the general arrangement of the hospital buildings on the site. (See Fig. 43.)

The cost of this hospital was £285 per bed, or, exclusive of site, £270 per bed, which must be regarded as very moderate for a brick-built hospital complying with the usual requirements. Its comparatively low cost is to be ascribed to the following circumstances:

1. The cost of the site was not excessive, and as sewers, a public water service, and gas were available, and the site adjoined a high road, expense on works of sewage disposal, water supply and lighting, and also on road-making, was avoided.

2. The district appears to be one in which the price of building is low.

3. The hospital, though substantially built and provided with essential requirements, is of a plain and simple design and ordinary materials, ornament and superfluities being dispensed with. The ward-blocks closely follow the Board's model plans, being unprovided with accessories, such as single-bed wards, which, however useful, add materially to the cost. The furniture is also very plain, costing only £22. 2s. per bed.

There is a central heating system which cost, including subways for pipes, £732, but it is claimed that with such a system

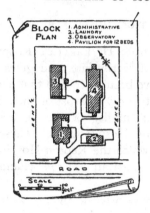

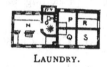

LAUNDRY.

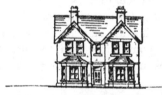

REPTON
ADMINISTRATIVE BLOCK—
FRONT ELEVATION.

LAUNDRY BLOCK.

———

—LAUNDRY.
—DRYING ROOM.
—INFECTED LINEN.
—DISINFECTED LINEN
—MORTUARY.
S—COAL.
T—W.C

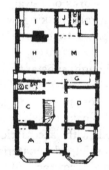

ADMINISTRATIVE BLOCK—
GROUND PLAN.

ADMINISTRATIVE BLOCK

A—MATRON'S ROOM.
B—MEDICAL ROOM.
C—STORE ROOM.
D—NURSES' ROOM.
E—W.C.
F—LAVATORY.
G—LARDER.
H—KITCHEN.
I—SCULLERY.
J—WOOD HOUSE.
K—SERVANTS W.C.
L—COAL HOUSE.
M—OPEN YARD.

SCALE—40 ft. = 1 in.

Fig. 41.   Showing plans of isolation hospital and administrative buildings at
Repton, Derbyshire.

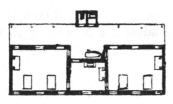

OBSERVATION BLOCK.
PLAN B OF L. G. B.

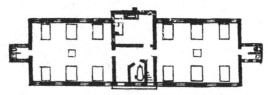

PLAN C OF L. G. B.
TWELVE-BEDDED PAVILION WITH TWO-BEDDED WARD ON FIRST FLOOR.

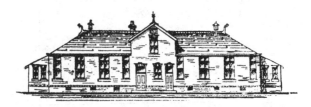

ELEVATION.

SCALE—40 ft. = 1 in.

Fig. 42. Showing plan and elevation of 12-bedded pavilion, with 2-bedded ward on first floor, of the Repton Isolation Hospital, and plan of observation block.

fewer and cheaper stoves suffice in the wards, and that it saves fuel, labour and dust; and that even when the ward-blocks are empty it is of advantage in enabling them to be kept dry, and in preventing damage to water pipes by freezing in cold weather.

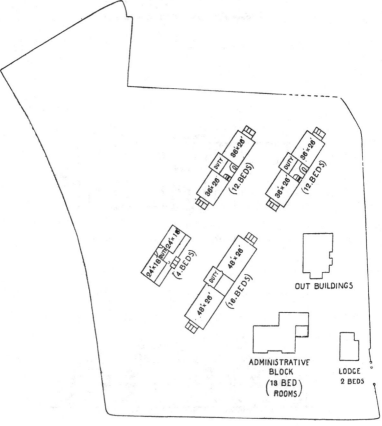

Fig. 43. Showing block plan of Stroud Joint Hospital Board's Infectious Diseases Hospital.

CHIDDINGSTONE JOINT ISOLATION HOSPITAL, KENT.

At this hospital the two ward-blocks, which are similar to one another, are of a special design here shown (see Fig. 44), each containing a 3-bed, a 2-bed, and a 1-bed ward; this design was

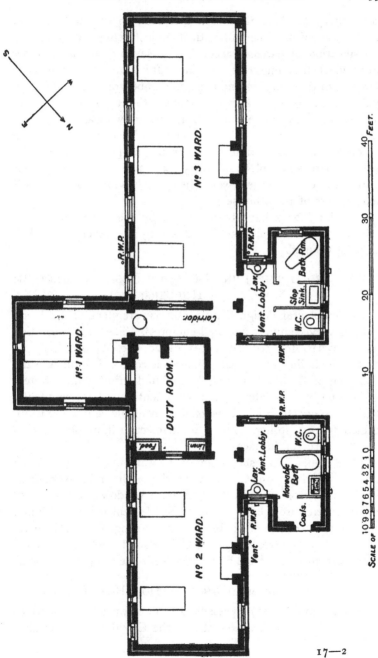

Fig. 44.   Showing plan of a ward-block at the Chiddingstone Joint Isolation Hospital.

planned by Mr Maberly Smith, architect, on the suggestion of Dr Tew, medical officer of health, its object being to facilitate the classification of patients according to sex and to the diseases from which they might be suffering. It is stated that experience has shown that varying and unequal numbers of male and female patients can be better accommodated without waste of space in a block of this arrangement than in one of two wards only. In a block with 3-bed, 2-bed and 1-bed wards, six patients can be accommodated at a time whatever the proportion of the two sexes, whereas in a block of two 3-bed wards if there were four patients of one sex, there would be no beds which could be used for patients of the other sex.

Similar blocks have been erected by the Sevenoaks Rural District at their hospital at Otford and by the Sevenoaks Urban District Council.

Colne and Holme Joint Isolation Hospital, Meltham Moor, near Huddersfield.

This hospital, designed by Mr Berry, architect, of Huddersfield, is very complete and well-equipped. The cost of erection was £23,310 for 50 bed-spaces of 2000 c. ft., or £466 per bed, or including site £484. The site is cold and bleak, and the warming of the wards having been found insufficient, a system of heating by hot-water pipes from a central underground boiler had to be constructed. Sewers were available, and water is obtained from a spring. There is an electric light plant and a small destructor furnace.

The plan, Fig. 45, shows one of the ward-blocks. It is based on the official plan C, but with the addition of verandahs approached from the wards by French windows, of single-bed wards entered from lobbies, and a convalescent room on the first floor over the centre of the block. The arrangement of the bathrooms in the annexes is ingenious. The single-bed wards and the convalescent rooms have been found very useful upon occasion.

Croydon Borough Isolation Hospital.

The plan (Fig. 47) represents a form of ward-block of which two have recently been erected by the Croydon Town Council

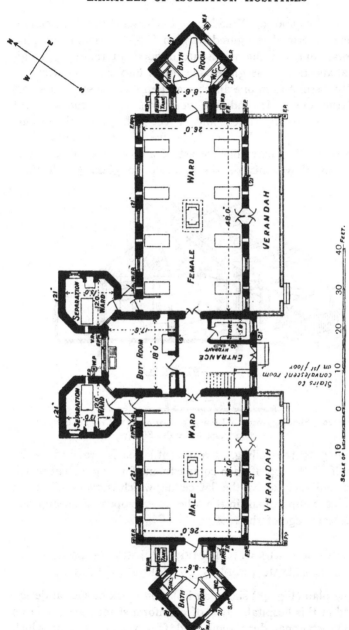

Fig. 45.   Colne and Holme Isolation Hospital.   Plan of a ward-block.

at their hospital at Waddon. Each ward-block resembles
in general form that figured in plan C of the Board's hospital
memorandum, but the wards are divided internally by longi-
tudinal and transverse glazed partitions into six compartments,
aerially distinct from one another and entered by separate doors
from the open air under a verandah. Each compartment
measures 12 feet by 12 feet and 11 feet in height to the ceiling,
and contains 1584 cubic feet, exclusive of the ventilating shaft
in the roof. The partitions consist of a dwarf wall about 3 feet
high, and, above this, of sheets of plate glass $\frac{1}{4}$-inch thick

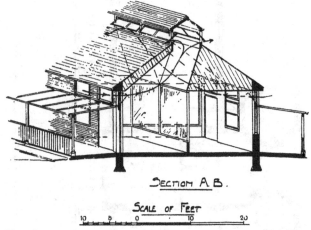

Section A B.

Scale of Feet

10   5   0   10   20

Fig. 46. Showing cross-ventilation of compartments at Croydon Borough
Isolation Hospital (see also Fig. 47).

extending to the ceiling. Cross ventilation is provided for by
one-half of the top of each compartment forming a shaft which
crosses obliquely above the flat ceiling which is over half of the
adjoining compartment in the other row, to open on the opposite
side of the ridge of the roof.

Croydon Rural and Merton Joint Isolation Hospital, Beddington Corner, Surrey.

The plan (Fig. 48) shows an isolation block of special design
erected at this hospital. It is of cruciform shape having a large
central octagonal duty room and four wings, each of which

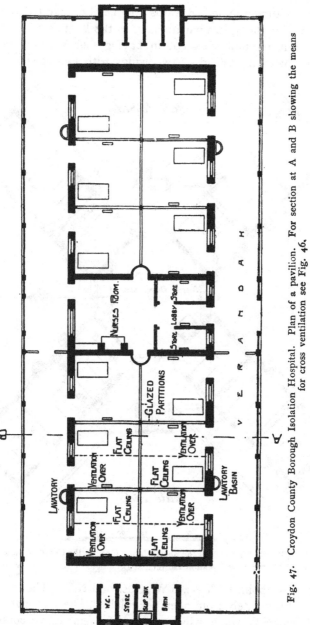

Fig. 47. Croydon County Borough Isolation Hospital. Plan of a pavilion. For section at A and B showing the means for cross ventilation see Fig. 46.

contains three single-bed wards completely separated from one
another by plate-glass partitions as in the Board's plan D, which
indeed it resembles, except in having four wings with three
rooms in each, instead of two wings with two rooms in each.

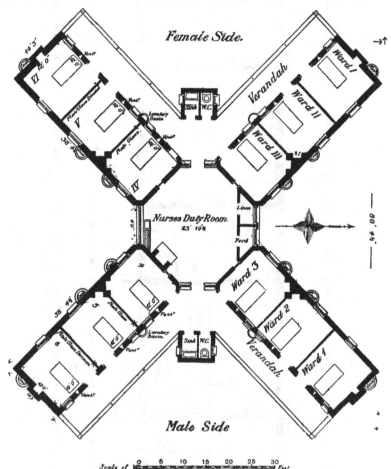

Fig. 48.   Showing plan of the new isolation block at the Croydon Rural and
Merton Joint Isolation Hospital at Beddington Corner, Surrey.

The wings point to N.W., S.W., S.E., and N.E.   The wards are
entered separately from open verandahs.   The verandahs of the
N.W. and S.W. wings, which are used for females, are continuous

with each other, meeting on the W. side at an angle in which is placed the annexe containing the w.c. and slop sink. The verandahs of the S.E. and N.E. wings, which are used for males, are similarly arranged. The area of each ward is 144 square feet, and its height 10 feet, giving 1440 cubic feet. There is one square foot of window area to each 70 cubic feet of space. The wards are warmed by fireplaces on the floor level, without grates. To each ward there is an external coal-bunker built of reinforced concrete, of hopper shape, opening by a door at the bottom into the ward at floor level close to the fireplace. This arrangement is said to effect a great saving of labour, as there is no need to carry coals into the wards; the bunkers are accessible to carts, and the carter, when delivering coals, has only to empty a sack into each bunker. There is a lavatory basin in each verandah, with two pedal-action taps, for hot and cold water respectively.

The experience of the new block is said to have been quite satisfactory; the nursing has not presented any difficulty, and there have been no cases of cross-infection. It is found convenient to place young children in the rooms nearest to the duty room.

The cost of this block, including drainage (£120), was £2195, or £183 per bed. The cost of the coal bunkers was £4. 7s. 6d. each, £52. 10s. in all. The block was therefore not a very expensive one, but it occupies a good deal of space on the ground.

KIRKBURTON JOINT ISOLATION HOSPITAL, NEAR HUDDERSFIELD.

The plan, Fig. 49, shows a pavilion on a modification of the Board's plan C, containing 18 beds in an 8-bed, a 6-bed, and two 2-bed wards; the latter are formed by partitioning off the ends of the ward-block, the sanitary annexes being placed at the sides of the block with entrances through a lobby from both the main and separation wards.

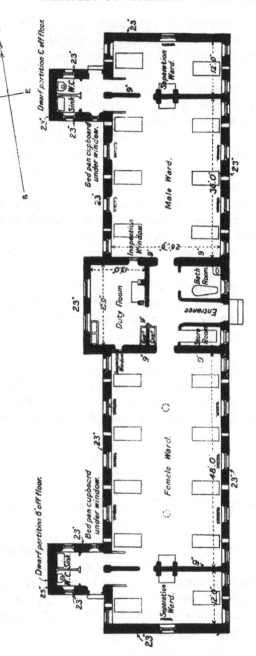

Fig. 49. Showing plan of a pavilion at the Kirkburton Joint Isolation Hospital.

LYDD ISOLATION HOSPITAL.

This is a small and cheap hospital, containing six beds in two wards, with nurses' accommodation, washhouse, etc., in a single block, deemed sufficient for a very small borough. The hospital is a two-storey building, and was designed by Mr Thurlow Fenn, architect, somewhat on the lines of the Local Government Board's former plan A, see Fig. 50.

SEDBERGH ISOLATION HOSPITAL.

This is a very small hospital, designed to meet a special case. The Sedbergh Rural District, which it serves, is an extensive and mountainous area of 52,665 acres, with a population under 4000 ; it contains however the small town of Sedbergh, at which there is an important grammar school. It was deemed necessary that there should be means for isolating infectious cases, but the district is an outlying one and remote from any more populous place with which a combination could be arranged. A separate hospital had therefore to be erected, but in view of the small population and resources of the district this had to be one on the smallest scale.

The hospital (see Figs. 51, 52 and 53) is on a modification of the former plan A of the Local Government Board, and contains on the ground floor two 2-bed wards and a kitchen, and on the first floor three bedrooms for nurses, approached by a staircase from the kitchen. There is a separate washhouse block on the lines of that in plan A. The hospital is built of local stone. Water is laid on from a public service, but sewage has to be treated on the site, which has an area of $1\frac{1}{4}$ acres and cost £250. The estimated cost of the hospital was £1296, or £324 per bed.

The plan might be useful for a sanatorium for a school or institution.

WALTHAMSTOW HOSPITAL.

The ward-block shown below, Fig. 54, is the first erected in this country on the principle of dividing the wards by glass partitions into separate compartments, each entered from the

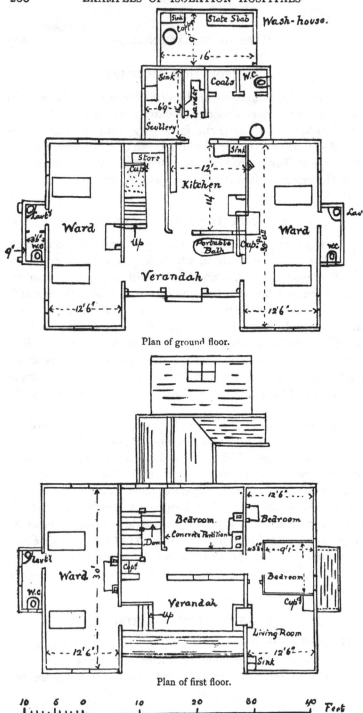

Plan of ground floor.

Plan of first floor.

Fig. 50. Borough of Lydd Isolation Hospital.

open air. The plan is similar to that of the isolation blocks at the Croydon Borough Hospital, but has not the overhead arrangement for cross-ventilation there shown.

Each compartment is heated by a radiator, and, besides a window of the usual hospital pattern, has four ventilating

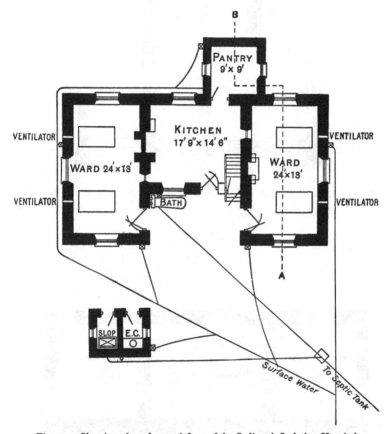

Fig. 51. Showing plan of ground floor of the Sedbergh Isolation Hospital.

openings as follows, the first two being intended as inlets and the other two as outlets:

1st. A perforated box on the floor to which air from the outside is brought from an opening near the ground level beyond the verandah on the opposite side of the block through

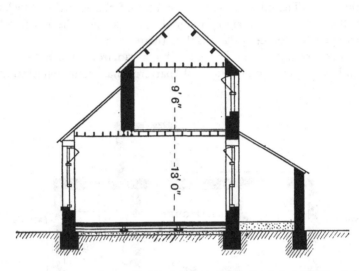

Fig. 52.   Section on line A—B of the building of the Sedbergh Isolation Hospital.

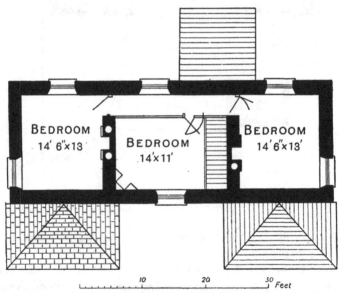

Fig. 53.   Showing plan of first floor of the Sedbergh Isolation Hospital.

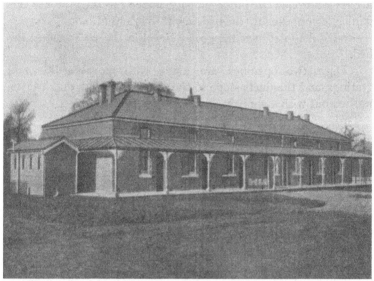

Fig. 54. Twelve-bed pavilion, showing separate door to each cubicle in the Walthamstow Isolation Hospital.

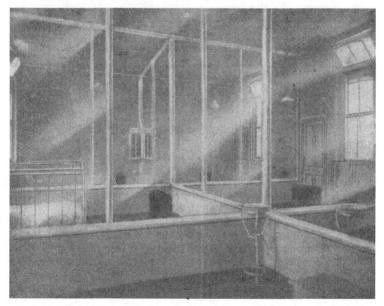

Fig. 55. Interior of pavilion, showing glass cubicles in the Walthamstow Isolation Hospital.

(The above illustrations are from the *Municipal Journal* of Feb. 16, 1906.)

a duct of stoneware pipes passing under the floor of the ad-joining compartment, thus giving through ventilation.

2nd.   An inlet near the ground level in the wall behind the bed.

(These two openings are made with movable lids and gratings, and the ducts slope to the outside, so that they can be washed out with a spray.)

3rd.   A Sheringham valve above the bed.

4th.   An opening in the ceiling.

Owing to the slope to the ground some of the inlets of the ducts have to be in pits below the ground level.

The lower illustration Fig. 55, shows how clear a view can be obtained from the duty-room inspection window, through the glass partitions, of the whole of the compartments in each half of the block.   Over each bed hangs an electric lamp which can be turned on by a switch in the duty-room (as well as by one in the verandah), so that the nurse, without leaving the duty-room, can get a view through the glass partitions of any patient in the block by lighting up his cubicle without lighting that of any other patient.   In the verandahs, by the door of each cubicle, are pegs for hanging overalls for the nurse and doctor, and there are also lavatory basins with push-taps delivering hot and cold water for their use.

BIBLIOGRAPHY

Thorne.   Hospital Report, 1882.   But see preface to reprint of 1901.
Parsons.   Hospital Report, 1912.
Barwise.   Report on the Isolation Hospitals of Derbyshire.   1906.

For illustrations and descriptions of other modern isolation hospitals reference may be made to series of articles in the *Public Health Engineer*, 1900–1901, and in the *Municipal Journal*, 1906, also to one of the Wimbledon isolation hospital in the *Surveyor and Municipal and County Engineer*, March 29, 1901, and to one of the Doncaster and Mexborough Joint Hospital at Conisborough in *The Hospital*, October 15, 1904.

INDEX